Acting Like an Animal

Playful Strengthening and Stretching Activities for Kid People

Tony Kemerly, Ph.D.

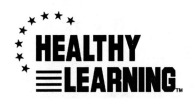

ISBN: 978-1-60679-176-9
Library of Congress Control Number: 2011928891
Cover design: Studio J Art & Design
Book layout: Studio J Art & Design
Front cover photo: PhotoObjects.net
Text photos: Trish Kemerly

Healthy Learning
P.O. Box 1828
Monterey, CA 93942
www.healthylearning.com

Dedication

This book is dedicated to my wife, Trish. Without her uncanny ability to see what is in my head and make it appear in a photograph, I don't know what I would do. Thank you for all of your support and patience.

Acknowledgments

Thanks to Deven and Elizabeth Snyder for being the most patient and physically skilled kids I could have hoped to use for this book. You have really set an example for kids everywhere. Thanks to Steve and Mariea Snyder for patiently waiting on me during the photo sessions and for helping to translate my instructions into "kid-speak."

Foreword

Tony Kemerly has created an exercise program designed to lead children through stretches that will help increase their flexibility and develop their overall muscular strength. The yoga-type poses in his book are presented through animals, which taps into a child's imagination and makes exercising fun. Animals are not only used for linking the image of the pose, but Kemerly also presents interesting facts about each animal, such as, "The horse's teeth occupy more room in its head than its brain."

Acting Like an Animal: Playful Strengthening and Stretching Activities for Kid People was written for teachers, coaches, parents, and other adults who work with children. I know they will find this to be a very creative manner in which to get children stretching. It is also written for the layperson who hasn't had formal training in exercise. The poses are visually displayed in photos and are accompanied by Activity Tips, written with easy-to-use language and definitions.

Another positive aspect of this program is that it can be presented in limited space areas. A teacher could actually scoot the classroom desk over, and the students can either participate all at once or take turns with different poses. Children's strength and flexibility has decreased with the overuse of computers, video games, and television, and it isn't enhanced by sitting in a classroom desk all day. These stretches can easily be done in a classroom for a few minutes, which will not only help the students' flexibility and strength, but also provide oxygen to the brain for better concentration with their studies.

I plan on using this in my university classes that prepare pre-service physical educators and elementary classroom teachers. I feel that it will be a strong addition to the other programs covered in the class, and will provide the teachers with an interesting way to present physical activity with animal facts.

—Martie Bell, Ph.D.
Associate Professor of Physical Education
High Point University

Past president for NCAAHPERD Physical Education Association
First elected committee chair for the National Association for Sport and Physical Education (NASPE)
P.E. steering committee coordinator for the High Point University Physical Education Teacher Education Program

Contents

    Effects of Obesity

        Physical Health

        Psychological Impact

    Causes of Obesity

        Genetics

        Environment: Diet and Leisure Habits

    Encouraging Children to Act Like an Animal

    Tortoise

    Opossum

    Mandrill

    Anteater

    Penguin

    Shrimp

    Mole

    Sidewinder

    Narwhal

    Lynx

    Rabbit

    Sitting Bear

    Inchworm

    King Cobra

    Flying Squirrel

    Catfish

1

Introduction

It is no secret that obesity is one of the major health concerns facing the country today. However, while most people's attention is directed toward the more well-known adult obesity crisis, the real problem is the uncontrolled rates of childhood obesity that are in part feeding the adult obesity epidemic. The numbers are staggering: 30 percent of children and adolescents from the ages of 6 to 19 are overweight, with 15 percent of those categorized as obese. The crux of the childhood obesity problem is that many people mistakenly separate childhood obesity from adult obesity, when in reality, one problem affects the other. The basis for this problem lies with the theory that a child will "grow out of" their obesity. This thinking is flawed and typically leads to an obese adolescent, and eventually, an obese adult. The reason for this is not what many parents think. It is not so much the excesses in diet or sedentary lifestyles; rather, it is the habits the children develop based on these behaviors that continue into adolescence and adulthood that cause this problem. Because of this, there is no chance for the child to grow out of their obesity because as they get older, these habits continue and typically worsen, resulting in adult obesity.

Effects of Obesity

Physical Health

The accumulation of excess body fat on a child will greatly affect the child's health. While all systems are affected by obesity, the major systems affected in children are the musculoskeletal, cardiovascular, and endocrine systems. Obesity affects a child's musculoskeletal system by placing it at great risk for serious structural problems such as decreased bone strength, an increased risk of fractures, osteoporosis, scoliosis, and even changes in the biomechanics of their walking gait[1-4]. A child's cardiovascular system is also affected by obesity by elevating the child's risk for heart disease as an adult[5-6]. Recent research indicates that obesity puts a child at risk for a case of "early atherosclerosis," or hardening of the arteries[7-8]. In addition to these problems, many other conditions that were previously thought to be "adult" cardiovascular problems, such as high blood pressure, are now being discovered in children[9]. A child's endocrine system is also affected by obesity through the development of Type II diabetes, which until the explosion of childhood obesity was a disease typically seen only in middle-aged adults[3]. Even more disturbing is the discovery of Insulin Resistance Syndrome or Syndrome X in children. Syndrome X, which was previously only found in adults, is a metabolic syndrome that combines hypertension, dyslipidemia, and insulin resistance[10]. Possibly two of the most disturbing aspects of childhood obesity are the increase in risk for adult obesity, as well as the parental influence on a child's risk of obesity. Research indicates that obese children are at a significantly higher risk of becoming obese adults. Furthermore, research also indicates that the risk is higher for becoming an obese adult if obesity was present during adolescence[11-14]. The physical effects of obesity are so severe that it is likely that this generation of children will reverse the trend of life expectancy and actually live shorter less healthy lives than their parents[15].

Psychological Impact

As if the physical ramifications of obesity were not troubling enough, the psychological effects of obesity are an insidious force, continuing throughout the adult life of the obese child. In fact, some research shows that the psychosocial factors of obesity are more detrimental than the physical symptoms[16]. It has been found that obese children are at an increased risk for depression, presumably as a result of childhood trauma related to the obesity[17-19]. These depressive symptoms, along with perceived social support from classmates and socioeconomic status, all have an effect on quality of life. Unfortunately for children, obesity negatively affects all of these factors, thereby leading to a great psychological impact on obese children[20-21]. Often, overweight children are excluded in social situations. This exclusion triggers a downward spiral for the child socially that coincides with low levels of self-esteem, which leads to a withdrawal from the social hierarchy by the child, resulting in diminished social skills, more behavioral problems, and lower self-images than normal weight children[22]. Another problem impacting obese children and adolescents is that of peer victimization. Peer victimization is an act of intentional aggression by a group of peers against someone they feel to be relatively weaker. These acts generally occur against individuals with low self-esteem, some degree of body dissatisfaction or social isolation, and/or a lack of psychosocial adjustment, all of which are traits found in obese children. Sadly, if the individual who is victimized does not possess these traits, the victimization typically results in the adoption of those behaviors[23]. In addition to enduring the physical abuses typical of peer victimization, overweight children are also at a greater risk to be the target of appearance-related teasing by peers as well as by siblings and even parents[24-27].

Causes of Obesity

As with any epidemic, childhood obesity has many factors that contribute to its rapidly expanding numbers. Generally, factors that cause childhood obesity are divided into two categories. Preventable risk factors are those that the child or parent can exercise some control over, such as physical activity level, diet, leisure time habits, or to some degree, their environment. The other type of risk factor is classified as non-preventable and includes the genetic component of the child and their family history.

Genetics

The genes inherited from parents and families are one small part of the obesity picture in children. Often, genes are thought to bind people to certain physical traits over which they have no control, but in the case of obesity that is not entirely true. While genes may predispose people to obesity, it must be understood that predisposition is not future fact. An individual predisposed to obesity will not become obese while engaging in daily exercise and eating a sensible diet. Predisposition implies that if the predisposed individual engages in unhealthy behaviors that have been shown to cause obesity, they will be more likely to become obese than someone who has no predisposition. The concept of predisposition implies that the true determinant of obesity is the interplay between genes and the environment[28]. Research indicates that genes play a relatively small role in the development of obesity, with between a 10 and 25 percent influence[29-30]. One of the primary reasons genetics are given credit for such a big role in the development of childhood obesity is because of the parent-child correlation. Research has shown that children of obese parents are at an increased risk for becoming obese themselves[31-34]. For example, a child with no obese parents has a 10 percent risk of becoming obese; if the child has one obese parent, the risk rises to 40 percent; and with two obese parents, the risk rises to 80 percent. The controversy arises when the reasoning for this disparity is hypothesized. Are children of obese parents more likely to be obese for purely genetic reasons, or is the environment the obese parent provides to blame?

Environment: Diet and Leisure Habits

The environment is considered by many to have a greater effect on childhood obesity than genetics. Environment is a powerful indicator for obesity as it consists of many different factors. For example, in the current climate, the issue of a child's diet is a controversial topic as it carries with it the implication of bad parenting. News stories depict parents who feed their children to excess as a way to keep them placated or as a reward for good behavior. The importance of a child's diet cannot be overstated, as recent research has shown us. One of the mistakes parents make with children is not educating them about their diet and the effect it will have on them. Parents mistakenly assume that children are unable to understand basic principles of healthy eating, so they make decisions based on what they feel is best for the child. However, research shows that the best dietary interventions for children include educating the child about the effects of their diet on their health[35]. Educating children about diet is important for two reasons: one, children spend a good deal of their time away from their parents and make at least one food decision on their own; and two, children are increasingly becoming a major target for junk-food advertisers[36]. Furthermore, education is needed, as it has been shown that parents who make unilateral decisions about their child's diet, rather than including the child in the decision-making process, are engaging in food restriction, which typically exacerbates their child's obesity[37]. When it comes to a child's diet, remember that the major problem with the eating habits of most children today is the amount of fat and sugar they typically eat on a daily basis. It is not just the fat- and sugar-laden foods that put them at great risk for developing obesity; it is also the sheer volume with which they are exposed to these foods from daycare, school lunches, or other supplemental meal programs[38-39]. It is unfair for the child to be educated in healthy diet options and not have the ability to make healthy choices. Decisions concerning a child's leisure time, however, are an entirely different matter.

Children's leisure time consists of what they do when not in school, participating in an extracurricular activity, or some other obligation. Leisure time activities have as much or more of an effect on the development of obesity in children than their diet. The primary leisure time activity that seems to be receiving the brunt of criticism from researchers for being a major cause of the obesity epidemic in children is watching television. The effect of children watching television has been studied with many different risk factors to determine its exact place in the childhood obesity epidemic. Unfortunately, many parents are not concerned with the amount of television their child watches[40] and do not realize that it is a much more complex factor in childhood obesity than was previously thought. It is more than just the sheer number of hours that cause the obesity; it is the exposure to advertisements for junk foods, which are often marketed expressly for children, as are the number of programs and commercials designed specifically for the child market. These child-centric advertisements number more than 40,000 per year, or over 100 per day[41-42]. An interesting point to note is a study that stated that children who watched more television typically ate fewer family meals. This decrease in family meals was correlated with a greater likelihood of being overweight[43]. This result is interesting in that it dovetails with other research that indicates that meals eaten away from the family are typically higher in fat and generally less healthy than family meals, which further reinforces the importance of the family meal[44]. Other research has shown that television watching during childhood establishes sedentary behavioral patterns that continue into adulthood, which result in greater instances of adult obesity[45-46]. Stopping the development of sedentary lifestyle habits is one of the most important steps in combating childhood obesity. The best way to combat these behaviors is to substitute them with another more positive behavior, in this case, physical activity.

Physical activity is an excellent method to battle childhood obesity, as it is a way to attack the problem by *adding* a fun activity that can be enjoyed by the entire family rather than *subtracting* an activity that is greatly enjoyed, such as food or television, resulting in a dislike of any new behavioral change. The research is clear in its conclusions: children who are physically active and do not engage in sedentary behaviors are protected against becoming overweight or obese[47-51]. Engaging in a physical activity program may be difficult for some in the beginning, as it requires a time commitment that some families may not have to give. However, the beauty of a physical activity program is that it can be done at anytime, and even in conjunction with other activities as a time-saver or as a counter-behavior to a negative habit. For example, many of the exercises in this book can be done while watching television. In this way, television can become a platform to develop healthy habits, such as being physically active, instead of using television time as an occasion to be sedentary and eat.

Encouraging Children to Act Like an Animal

When it comes to children, parents often wish to protect them from anything that could cause them harm. While this mind-set is necessary and unfortunately required in this day and age, regrettably, it has filtered into the physical activity patterns of children. Children today are either not allowed or do not have access to unsupervised play with other children in the neighborhood. While this approach was the norm just 20 years ago, today, the physical activity level of a child is dependent upon the parent's ability to drive them to a facility in which their activity program is housed. This dependence, combined with the ever-increasing number of families in which both parents work, results in a parent not necessarily being available to take a child to a dance or martial arts class or a sports practice session. Instead, either the child receives less physical activity at an afterschool program that is typically underfunded and understaffed, or in the worst-case scenario, the child does not get any physical activity at all.

This book is designed to provide a series of exercises that can be done anywhere, anytime, and anyplace, without the need for any equipment and with small requirements for space. The exercises are categorized in a few ways: first, they are arranged according to the parts of the body that are stretched or strengthened by the exercise; second, they are arranged within the anatomical foci by level of difficulty; and third, they are arranged in a pattern that allows the movements to flow from one to the next. Finally, at the end of the book is an appendix of sample exercise programs that provide a plan to follow during exercise sessions. The exercises present enough of a challenge that anyone in the family can join in.

2

Back and Abdominal Exercises

The back muscles are among the most important set of muscles in the entire body. Many people overlook both the importance and number of muscles that are found in the back. The arrangement of the muscles of the back is such that one layer is on top of another, which is on top of another. At the deepest levels, the intertransversarii muscles help with movements that may occur between individual vertebrae. In contrast, the multifidus muscle aids in moving the spine as a single unit. On top of those are the erector spinae, which are helpful in maintaining good posture. Finally, the most superficial layer of back muscles, which include the trapezius, is involved with moving the neck or shoulder girdle. These muscles help to move the entire back in relation to the rest of the body. The proper functioning of these muscles is important as the back provides support for the head as well as the trunk of the body. The back has a tough job in that not only does it have to be strong, but it also has to be flexible enough to allow you to move through a large range of motion. It is important for children to have strong, supple backs so that they can avoid dealing with lower back pain, which is the most common type of pain endured by adults. Unfortunately, the back muscles are often ignored until a problem occurs. This is likely due to the fact that people do not realize how involved the back muscles are in their daily lives. Sneezing, breathing, sitting, standing, bending, twisting, reaching, and carrying motions all rely on a healthy back to be performed pain-free. There is a saying about the back: "A healthy back is the key to a healthy body." A truer statement could not be said, as having a healthy back is one of the keys to having a full, active life.

The abdominal muscles are typically referred to as "the core." The four muscles generally mentioned when referring to the abdominal muscles are the rectus abdominis, external oblique, internal oblique, and the transverse abdominis. The rectus abdominis is the most well-known of the abdominal muscles, as it is responsible for the sought-after "six pack" found in many lean individuals. While the rectus abdominis is responsible for flexing the trunk (pulling the chest downward), its importance as a muscle for posture should not be overlooked. The oblique muscles, internal and external, are also responsible for flexion of the trunk, but do so with a rotational flair, meaning when they contract, they tend to turn the body toward the side of that particular muscle. Finally, the transverse abdominis, while often overlooked since it is not a superficial muscle and therefore is not seen, is quite important as a core stabilizer, as it acts as the body's natural "weight belt" when attempting to lift a heavy object. The importance of the abdominal muscles as a group is their role as a connection between the upper and lower body. If the body is viewed as a three-link chain, the abdominal muscles are that important middle link in the chain. Finally, because the abdominal muscles work in tandem with many of the intrinsic muscles of the back that were previously mentioned, strong, healthy abdominal muscles are an important component of a strong, healthy back.

Tortoise

Animal Facts:

- The desert tortoise lives in an area where the temperature reaches 140 degrees Fahrenheit.
- The record for the world's largest tortoise is a Galapagos tortoise that was two feet tall, almost three-and-a-half feet wide, nearly 54 inches long, and weighed 900 pounds.
- The oldest living animal on the planet is a 175-year-old tortoise.

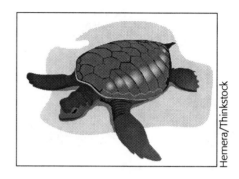

Hemera/Thinkstock

Activity Tips:

- The goal is to keep the forehead on the floor.
- The hips should remain level, and the buttocks should sit back between the heels.
- The knees may be opened a little if it becomes difficult to breathe.

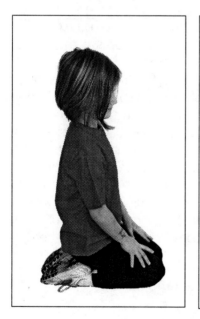
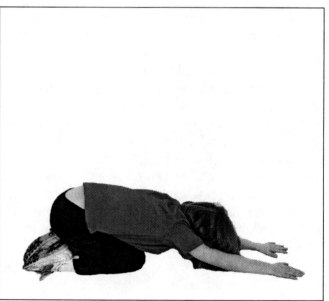

Opossum

Animal Facts:

- When it is frightened and unable to run, it goes into an involuntary shock where it appears dead.
- Opossums have 50 teeth, more than any North American land mammal; and they use them for climbing.
- Opossums lived over 70 million years ago during the age of the dinosaurs.

Activity Tips:

- The goal is to keep the forehead on the floor.
- The hips should remain level, and the buttocks should sit back between the heels.
- As much of the top of the thigh (of the leg that is extended backward) as is possible should be in contact with the floor.

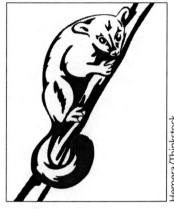

Hemera/Thinkstock

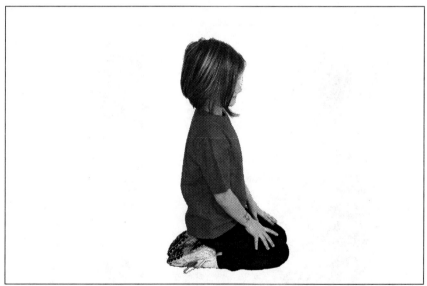

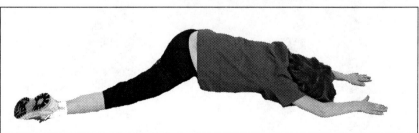

Mandrill

Animal Facts:

- The mandrill is the world's largest monkey, with the male about two-and-a-half feet tall and about 100 pounds.
- Mandrills are well known for the colorful faces that range in color from bright reds and purples to blue; the front ends even match the back ends.
- The colors on a male's face become more apparent when he is threatening lower ranking members of his group.

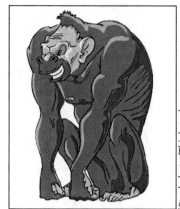

iStockphoto/Thinkstock

Activity Tips:

- The heels should be flat on the ground, if at all possible.
- The arms and torso should rest between the legs.
- The weight of the body, rather than a bouncing movement, should be used to complete the stretch.

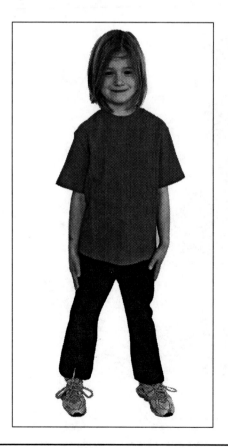

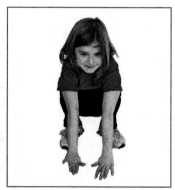

Front view

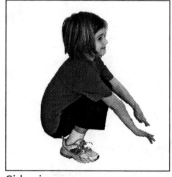

Side view

Anteater

Animal Facts:

- An anteater is nearly six feet long, but its mouth is only an inch wide.
- Anteaters will not completely destroy a nest; instead, they will eat only a few thousand ants, let them recover, and go back for more.

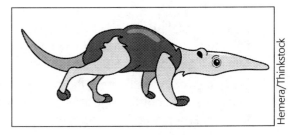

- The anteater has a sticky, two-foot long tongue that it can flick in and out 60 times per minute.

Activity Tips:

- Firm contact needs to be maintained between the feet and the ground.
- The navel should be pushed upward toward the ceiling.
- The goal is to keep the spine and neck straight while keeping the chin off the chest.

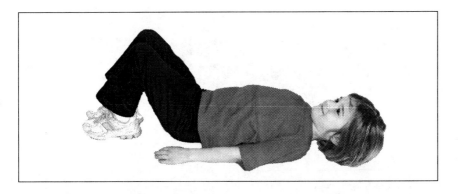

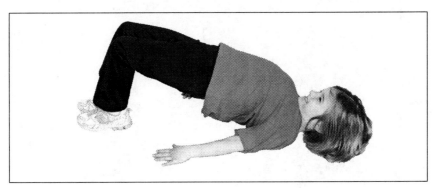

Penguin

Animal Facts:

- Penguins are the only bird that can swim and not fly. The largest, the Emperor Penguin, can grow to four feet tall and weigh 90 pounds.
- Penguins mate for life with the mother and father penguins sharing responsibility for hatching, feeding, and protecting their young.
- Penguins use a type of sign language to communicate which consists of waving their flippers and moving their heads.

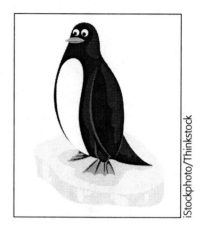

iStockphoto/Thinkstock

Activity Tips:

- The goal is to roll the knees into the chest before pushing them up to the ceiling.
- The spine and neck should be kept straight while keeping the chin off the chest.
- In the final position, the weight should be off the neck, and the head should not turn from side to side.

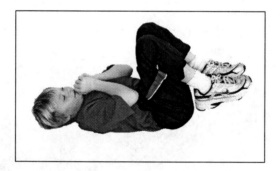

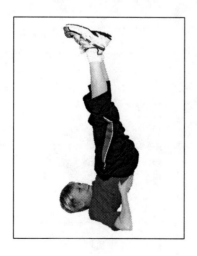 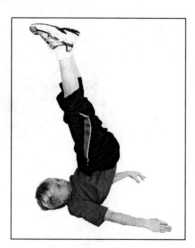

Shrimp

Animal Facts:

- A shrimp's heart is located inside its head.
- The world's largest shrimp was nearly 16 inches long.
- A mantis shrimp is able to snap its claws shut at the speed of a .22 caliber bullet.

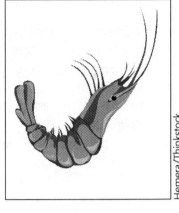
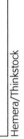

Activity Tips:

- From Penguin, the knees should be bent toward the chest before moving into Shrimp.
- The back should be kept as straight as possible while the toes are lowered to the ground.
- While in the final position, the weight should be kept off the neck, and the head should not turn from side to side.

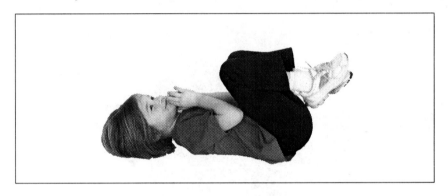

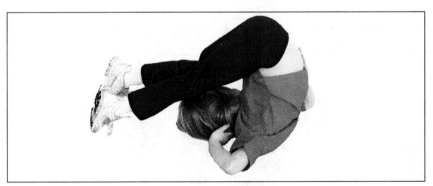

Mole

Animal Facts:

- The tentacles on the star-nosed mole are the most sensitive sensory organ of any mammal.
- The shrew mole only sleeps eight minutes at a time and then stays awake for a maximum of 18 minutes before falling asleep again.
- Moles have a large appetite and eat between 80 and 100 percent of their weight in food each day.

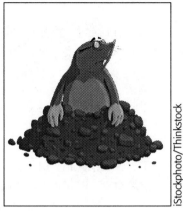

iStockphoto/Thinkstock

Activity Tips:

- Comfort in Shrimp should be achieved before attempting Mole.
- The spine will round a little during this exercise, but again, the weight should be kept off the neck, and the head should not turn from side to side.
- Normal breathing should be followed throughout the exercise.

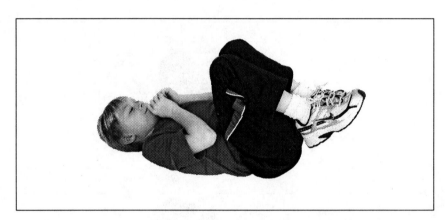

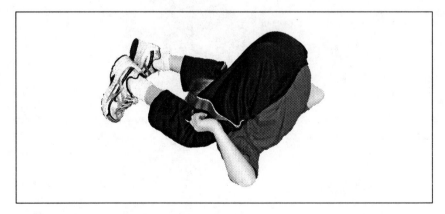

Sidewinder

Animal Facts:

- Sidewinder is a common name for a rattlesnake.
- Sidewinders move in their looping fashion so that they can get traction on sandy surfaces and to avoid being overheated by the sand, as only three points touch the ground at a time.
- Sidewinders are often called horned rattlesnakes because they have a small horn over each eye.

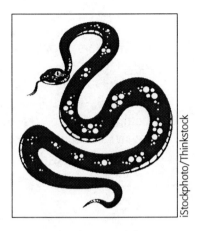

iStockphoto/Thinkstock

Activity Tips:

- Before moving, the goal is to lift the body off the ground with the feet and core muscles.
- While the body will be moving in many directions, the path should be that of a straight line.
- Each repetition should be finished with the hands touching the toes.

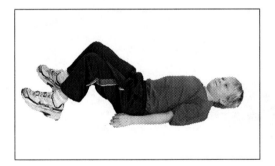
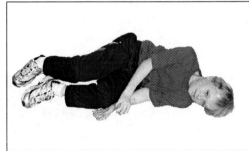
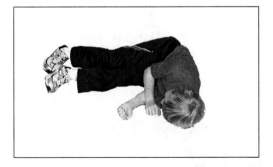
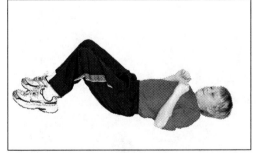

Narwhal

Animal Facts:

- Narwhals are known as the unicorns of the sea as they have a tusk that extends eight to nine feet from their heads.
- Their tusk, which is actually an elongated tooth, always projects from the left side of the jaw and spirals to the left.

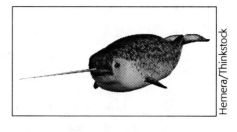

Hemera/Thinkstock

- Narwhal is an Old Norse word meaning "corpselike." Narwhals are so named because of their mottled black, white, and greenish coloring.

Activity Tips:

- The back should not arch. The focus should be kept on pushing the lower back into the floor.
- In order to maintain balance, the arms may be extended over the head.
- The exercise may be modified for ease by putting the hands under the hips.

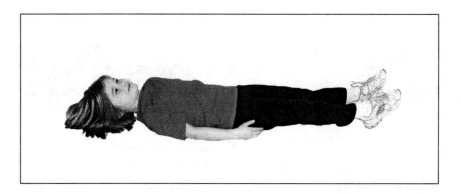

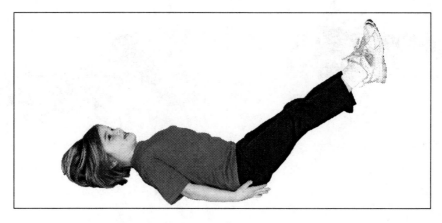

Lynx

Animal Facts:

- While it averages only about 25 pounds in size, the lynx is a ferocious and dangerous hunter.
- Because the lynx spends so much time in the snow, the feet are very large and act like snowshoes. For example, a 30-pound lynx has bigger feet than a 200-pound mountain lion.
- While they are often mistaken for bobcats, lynx have tufts of fur on tops of their ears, giving them a pointed appearance.

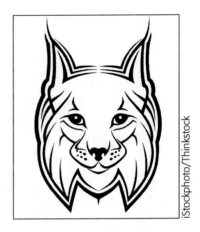

iStockphoto/Thinkstock

Activity Tips:

- The back should only arch as much as necessary.
- The position of the arms and legs may vary.
- The focus should be on normal breathing throughout the movement.

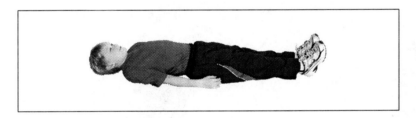

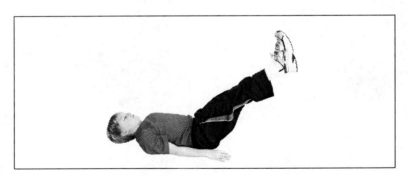

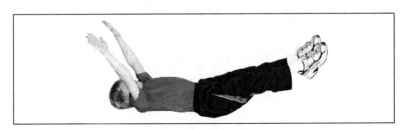

Rabbit

Animal Facts:

- Rabbits are able to see behind them without turning their heads, but have a blind spot in front of their face.
- Groups of rabbits called herds live inside a warren, which is set up much like a human's house. The warren includes rooms for sleeping, rooms for babies (kits), and even restrooms.
- When rabbits are happy, they will jump in the air and twist; this is known as a binky.

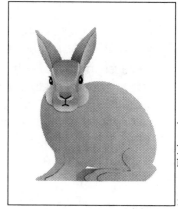

Hemera/Thinkstock

Activity Tips:

- Each individual should be allowed time to find a balance point.
- Once balance is achieved, the abs should be tightened to hold position.
- The position of the arms and legs can vary.

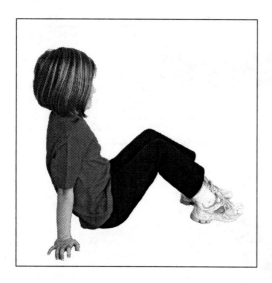
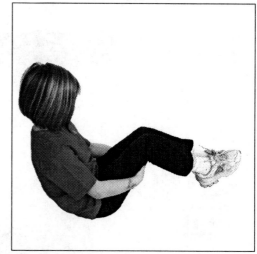

Sitting Bear

Animal Facts:

- A grizzly bear can run as fast as the average horse, about 45 mph.
- All polar bears are left-handed.
- At birth, a panda bear is smaller than a mouse.

Activity Tips:

- The knees most likely will bend when the first attempt at straightening the legs is made.
- Each individual should be allowed time to find a balance point.
- The goal is to move the legs as far apart as possible.

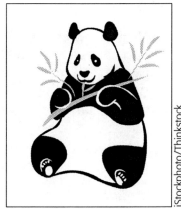

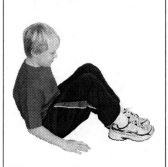
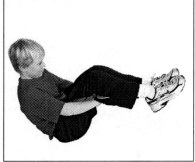

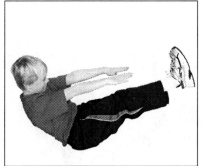
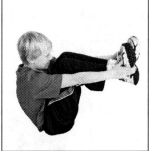
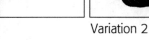

Variation 1   Variation 2

Inchworm

Animal Facts:

- Many inchworms have odd projections on their bodies that are meant to resemble small twigs, thereby making them hard to see.
- When threatened, some inchworms will stand straight up on a branch so that they can resemble a twig.
- Inchworms are not worms at all, but larvae that will soon become moths.

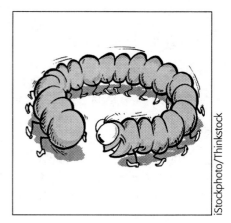

iStockphoto/Thinkstock

Activity Tips:

- The hands should be used at a slow and even pace to lower the body forward toward the ground.
- The feet should then move toward the hands at the same pace.
- The hands should continue to move forward until the body is as close to parallel to the ground as possible.

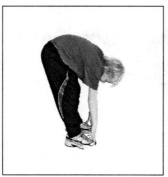
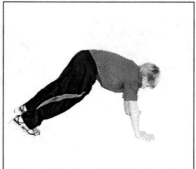

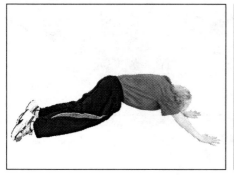
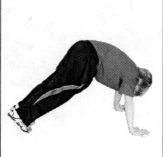
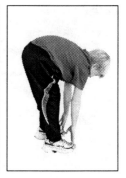

King Cobra

Animal Facts:

- The king cobra is the largest venomous snake and is considered to be the most intelligent.
- They can grow to 18 feet in length and weigh 200 pounds and are capable of looking you in the eyes by "standing up."
- The amount of venom the king cobra injects with each bite is toxic enough to kill an elephant or 20 men.

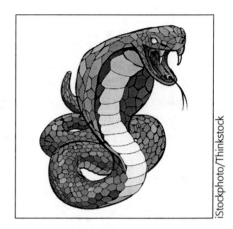

iStockphoto/Thinkstock

Activity Tips:

- The palms should be flat on the floor beneath the shoulders.
- The focus should be on pressing the toenails firmly into the mat to aid in balance.
- Slow movement and an elongated spine should be encouraged; the head should not be thrown back as far as possible.

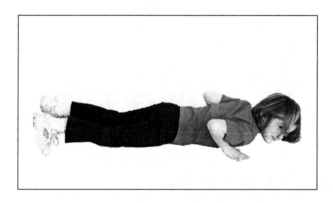

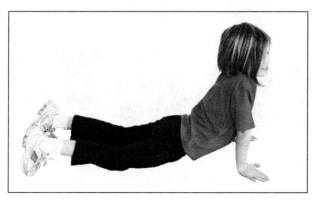

Flying Squirrel

Animal Facts:

- These squirrels do not actually fly, but instead they glide and are capable of doing so for distances of over 100 feet.
- They can glide because of a large fold of skin called a patagium between the front and rear feet that acts as a parachute when they leap from trees.
- Because they hunt at night, they have large "bug" eyes to allow them to see well.

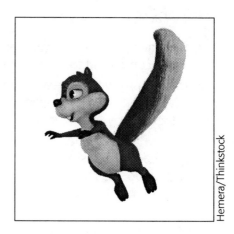

Hemera/Thinkstock

Activity Tips:

- The body must remain tight throughout the exercise.
- The goal should be to get as long as possible by reaching forward with the arms and backward with the legs.
- The waist should be the only point of contact with the ground.

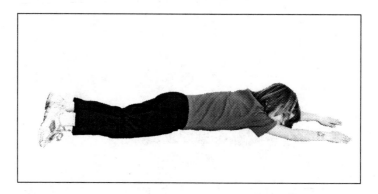

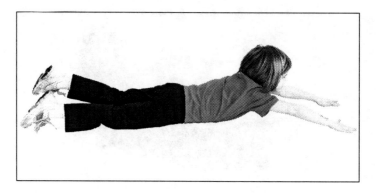

Catfish

Animal Facts:

- The largest catfish ever caught was in Russia; it was 16.5 feet long and weighed 660 pounds.
- Catfish have over 27,000 taste buds, which are more than is possessed by any other animal.
- The glass catfish is almost completely transparent, meaning that you can see through it.

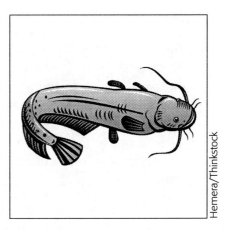

Hemera/Thinkstock

Activity Tips:

- The foot should be pulled up toward the ceiling, not toward the head.
- Balance will be improved by keeping good contact with the ground.
- The focus should remain on keeping an elongated spine throughout the movement.

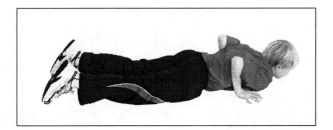

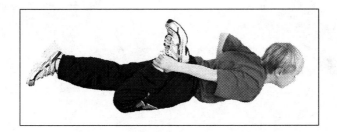

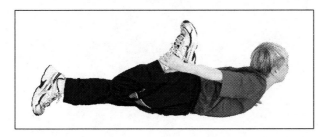

Tiger

Animal Facts:

- Tiger stripes are as individual as human fingerprints.
- All tigers have a similar mark on their foreheads; this mark resembles the Chinese symbol for king.
- Like housecats, tigers have retractable claws; however, unlike housecats, tigers love to swim.

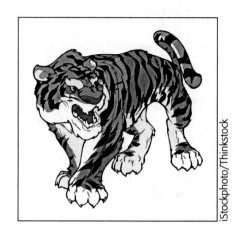

iStockphoto/Thinkstock

Activity Tips:

- The back should be kept as straight and as long as possible.
- The foot should be pulled up toward the ceiling, not the back of the head.
- The goal is to look up, but the head should not fall backward; the neck should stay straight.

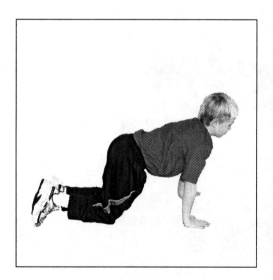
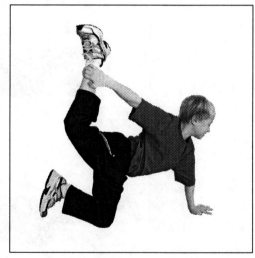

Puffer Fish

Animal Facts:

- When angry or threatened, puffer fish "puff" themselves up to appear bigger to other fish; some even puff up and have spines sticking off of them.
- One type of puffer, a fugu, has a powerful toxin in its organs that must be removed before eating or death will occur.
- Sharks are generally one of the few fish to attempt to eat a puffer fish.

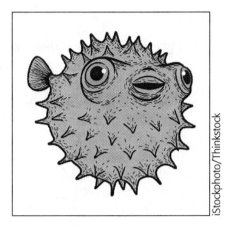

iStockphoto/Thinkstock

Activity Tips:

- The goal is to lift the chest while performing the movement.
- The feet should pull the hands in an upward direction. It is a pulling motion of the arms and legs, not a crunching of the back.
- To increase difficulty, an effort should be made to keep the knees together throughout the movement.

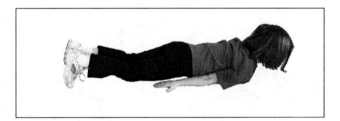

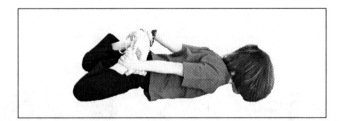

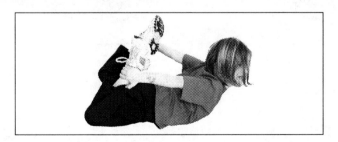

Ankylosaurus

Animal Facts:

- An adult was about 30 feet long, six feet wide, six feet tall, and could weigh four tons with a back completely covered in spiny armor.
- It had a club-like tail that it used to protect itself from other dinosaurs like the Tyrannosaurus rex.
- The ankylosaurus is a popular dinosaur that is often compared to a living tank.

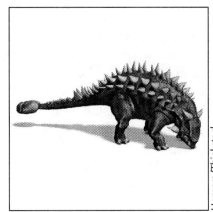

Hemera/Thinkstock

Activity Tips:

- The chest lift off the floor and foot lift should be done simultaneously.
- Breath holding should be discouraged, as it will make the movement more difficult. Normal breathing throughout the movement should be the goal.
- As with the Puffer Fish, the foot is pulled up toward the ceiling, not forward toward the head.

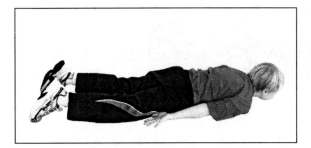

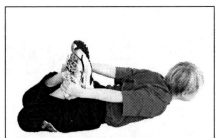

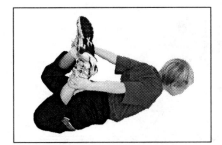

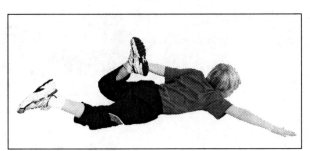

Eel

Animal Facts:

- Eels can swim forward and backward, and can live out of the water for up to 48 hours.
- Electric eels can grow to be eight feet long and emit a pulse of 500 volts.
- Moray eels are extremely vicious and will often not let go of a victim once it bites.

Activity Tips:

- The focus should be on pushing the chest forward and the navel upward during the exercise.
- The back may be supported during the movement, if necessary.
- When exiting the position, the head should first be brought to the floor, and then the hips lowered.

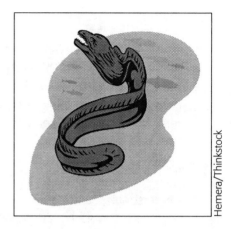

Hemera/Thinkstock

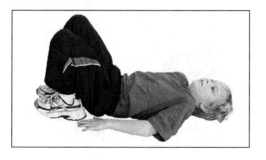 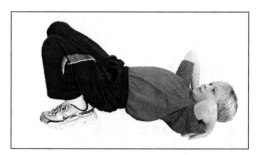

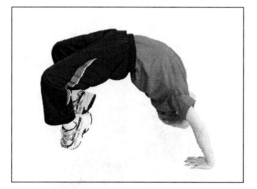

Gecko

Animal Facts:

- Geckos can stick to walls as a result of tiny barbed hairs that protrude from their feet.
- Some geckos have skin that feels like velvet.
- Some geckos have folds of skin that prevent them from having a shadow, which keeps them safe from predators.

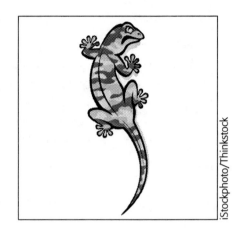

Activity Tips:

- Interpersonal competition during this movement should be discouraged. The goal is to move slowly and only as far as the body allows.
- The end goal of the movement is to look under the armpit to the ceiling.
- Comfort in Eel is a prerequisite for attempting Gecko.

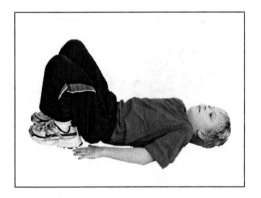 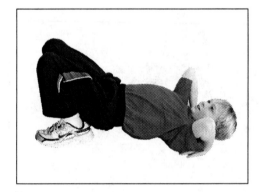

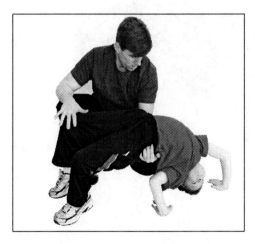

Shark

Animal Facts:

- A shark has excellent hearing—so good, in fact, that it finds fish to eat by hearing their heartbeat.
- A shark does not have a single bone in its body; its entire skeleton is made of cartilage.
- Sharks will eat anything; case in point, the following have been found inside a shark's stomach: nails, a bottle of wine, a treasure chest, a suit of armor, license plates, a drum, and even a torpedo.

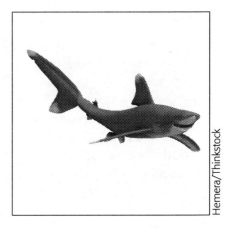

Hemera/Thinkstock

Activity Tips:

- As a straight leg is the goal of the movement, focus should remain on that aspect, rather than on how high the leg can be lifted.
- Balance will likely be an issue, so the focus should remain on keeping the abs tight throughout the movement.
- To exit the movement safely, the leg should be brought down before bringing the body to the floor, as in Eel.

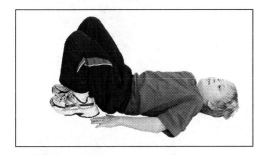
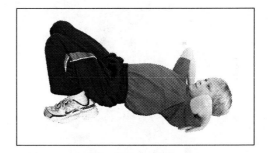
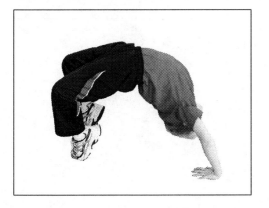
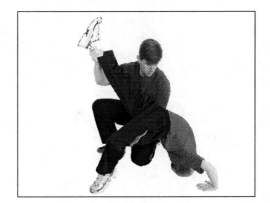

Click Beetle

Animal Facts:

- The "click" is used as a way for the beetle to right itself if stuck on its back or to avoid predators.
- They are skilled at "thanotosis," or faking death to avoid predators, and will roll up their antenna and curl their legs close to their body for a long time.
- Some have large false eyes on their backs as a way to scare off predators.

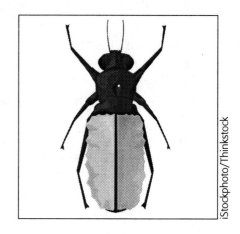

iStockphoto/Thinkstock

Activity Tips:

- In order to maintain support and still remain balanced, the arms should be kept firm, but focus should remain on supple hips to allow movement.
- The movement should be initiated by moving one leg under the body to turn over.
- A bend in the arms may be necessary to complete the turn.

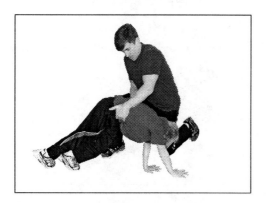
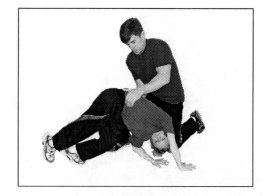
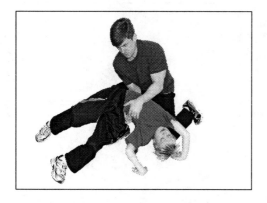
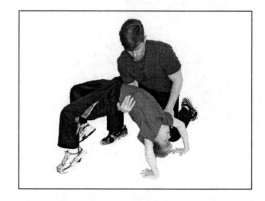

Tarantula

Animal Facts:

- Tarantulas are the largest of the spiders, with some measuring up to a foot in length.
- Tarantulas do not spin a web to catch prey; instead, they get their food by chasing it down and biting it.
- A tarantula's hairy coat and sensitive feet help it to find prey.

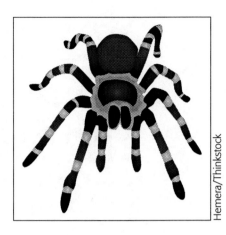

Hemera/Thinkstock

Activity Tips:

- The head should be kept in a position that allows the child to see where he is moving.
- The arms and legs should move contralaterally. If they do not, a loss of balance will likely occur.
- Slow, steady movement is the goal when learning this movement. A move should only occur when balance is established in the previous position.

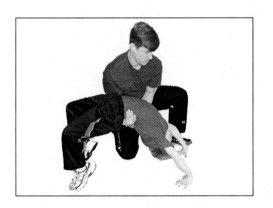
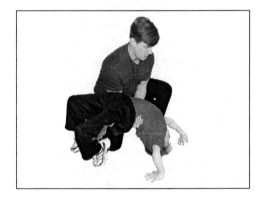

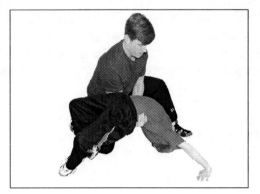

3

Hip and Leg Exercises

The muscle group known as the hamstrings consists of the *semimembranosus*, *semitendinosus*, and the *biceps femoris*. Their purpose is twofold: they assist the *gluteus maximus* in extending the hip, and they are the primary group of muscles responsible for flexing the knee. As such, they are quite active during movements such as walking, running, and jumping. Unfortunately, the hamstrings are one of the most overlooked groups of muscles of the lower extremity. Ideally, a 3:1 ratio of strength should exist between the quadriceps and the hamstrings; meaning, if a person can lift 100 pounds on the seated leg extension, he should be able to lift 35 pounds on the leg curl machine. Maintenance of this ratio is important because the hamstrings act as the "brake" for straightening or extending the knee while sprinting. When this ratio is higher, the hamstrings become more at risk of injury. It is this type of injury to the hamstrings, known as a "pulled hamstring," that is the most common. Flexibility of the hamstrings is important not only for the reason mentioned, but also because tightness in the hamstrings is often associated with a variety of conditions, from lower back pain to poor posture to misalignment of the pelvis. Unfortunately, hamstring inflexibility is rampant today as a result of the lack of use of this muscle group. Because people do not spend much time sitting on the ground or bending over repeatedly, and instead spend time sitting in chairs, the hamstrings have suffered. The exercises in this chapter will serve to both strengthen and stretch the hamstrings, which will aid in preventing injury. Lastly, improvement in these exercises will also provide an increase in performance for some of the back exercises in Chapter 2.

The quadriceps muscle group is the most powerful group of muscles of the lower extremity. The quadriceps is comprised of four individual muscles: the *rectus femoris*, the *vastus medialis*, the *vastus intermedius*, and the *vastus lateralis.* Research indicates that having an appropriate level of quadriceps strength will help individuals by increasing balance, reducing knee pain, and avoiding injuries to the anterior cruciate knee ligament. Because of the overall mass of the quadriceps and its profound strength, the quadriceps is often susceptible to tightness or a lack of flexibility. Muscle tightness in the quadriceps can lead to tightness in the flexors of the hip as well, which can have an effect on posture. The importance of quadriceps strength lies in its importance as a foundational lower extremity muscle. The quadriceps provide an individual with a base of strength that is required for everything from dynamic exercises, such as running, kicking, and jumping, to basic activities of daily living like walking, standing from a seated position, or getting into or out of a car. Without a good level of strength of the quadriceps all of those actions become problematic and, in worst-case scenarios, dangerous due to a lack of balance.

The last set of muscles targeted by this group of exercises is the muscles of the hip. The group of hip muscles includes the *iliopsoas*, *rectus femoris*, *pectineus*, *sartorius*, and *tensor fascia latae*. These muscles are collectively known as the hip flexors and allow people to forcefully pull the thigh up toward the abdomen. The need to build strength and flexibility in the hip flexors comes from the fact that people sit in chairs most of the day. The seated position often results in tightness of the hip flexors, which can result in poor posture and lower back pain. Another group of muscles targeted by these exercises include the *adductor magnus*, *adductor longus*, *adductor brevis*, and the *gracilis*. These muscles, collectively known as the adductors, are needed to pull the leg back toward the body. The importance of the hip adductors is that they provide the ability to have good side-to-side agility, something needed to excel in most sports.

Lion

Animal Facts:

- A male lion's roar can be heard over five miles away.
- Lions do not hunt for their food, the lionesses hunt in packs for it.
- Lions can run up to 35 mph and jump over 30 feet.

Activity Tips:

- The goal is to focus on a straight-backed posture in this exercise while keeping the eyes forward.
- The body should be moved into the final position by lowering the body until the buttocks are resting on the heels.
- The goal is to let the body relax and sink into the position and avoid "holding up" the body while in the position.

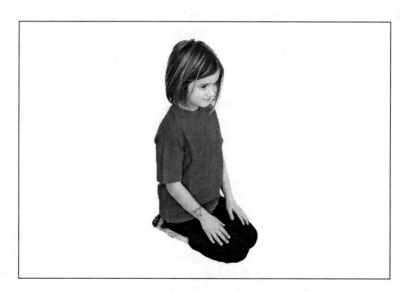

Horse

Animal Facts:

- A horse's teeth occupy more room in its head than its brain.
- One of the earliest horses was called a hyracotherium and only grew to the size of a fox.
- Horses communicate how they feel by using facial expressions.

Activity Tips:

- The hips must be pushed forward throughout the movement to maintain stability.
- The abdominal muscles must be relaxed in order to bend backward.
- Movement should be slow and steady, as this position may be unnatural to some participants.

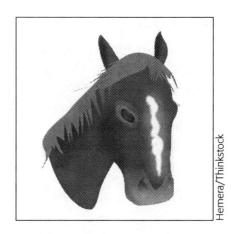

Hemera/Thinkstock

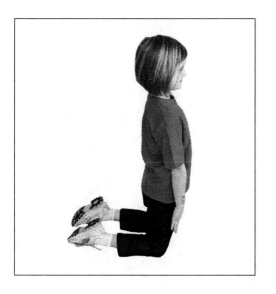
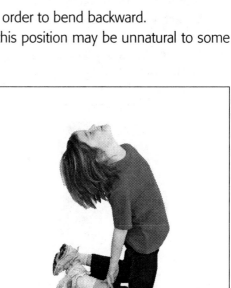

Camel

Animal Facts:

- Camels have a very thin third eyelid that they are able to see through which helps keep sand out of their eyes.
- A camel's hump is filled with fat. The hump shrinks when the camel does not eat.
- A camel is able to drink 27 gallons of water in 10 minutes.

Activity Tips:

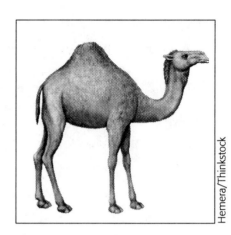

Hemera/Thinkstock

- The hips must be pushed forward throughout the movement to maintain stability.
- A variety of hand positions on the feet, back, heels, or knees should be encouraged.
- If the thighs are perpendicular to the ground throughout the exercise, the hips should be pushed forward.

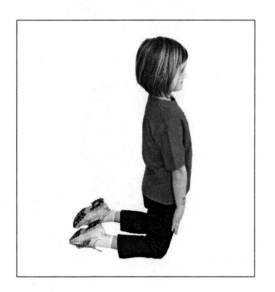
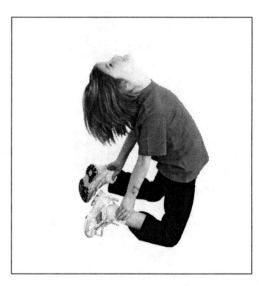

Roly-Poly

Animal Facts:

- The roly-poly, or pill bug, is not a bug, but rather an arthropod, meaning it is related to crawfish, crabs, and shrimp.
- They do not sting, bite, or pinch; instead, they roll up into a tight ball when they feel threatened.
- They are the only crustacean to move onto the land with a great amount of success.

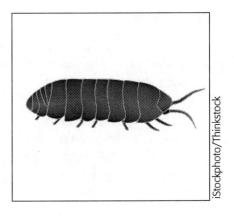

iStockphoto/Thinkstock

Activity Tips:

- The knees should point upward throughout the exercise.
- For smooth movement into position, a good grip should be kept on the front of the legs during the backward lean.
- The movement will finish by curling up toward the knees, as if doing a sit-up.

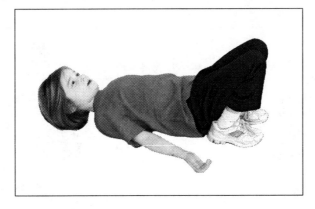

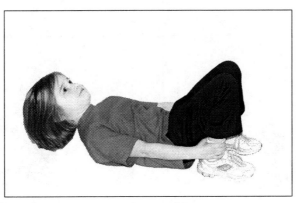

Duck

Animal Facts:

- Ducks have a gland near the tail that secretes an oil onto their feathers, thereby making their feathers waterproof.
- Ducks get food from below the surface by "dabbling," or sticking their heads under water with their tails pointing straight up in the air.
- Ducks use their beaks for scooping food out from the bottom of a pond.

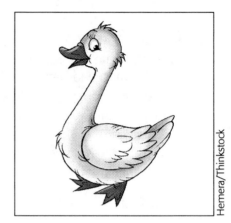

Activity Tips:

- The movement can easily be varied for intensity by changing the direction of movement.
- The hands should not touch the ground throughout the movement. Doing so will result in sloppy movement.
- A slight bouncing motion of the body will likely accompany this movement.

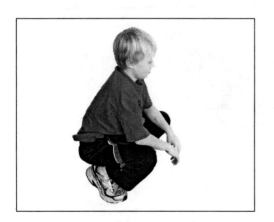
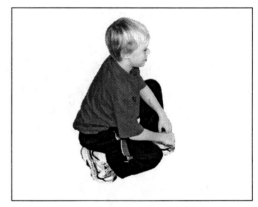
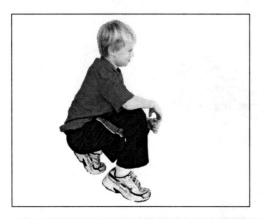
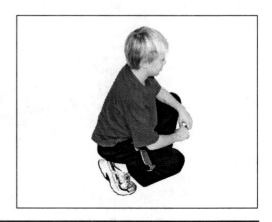

Meerkat

Animal Facts:

- Meerkats are extremely social animals, so much so that when a predator attacks, the group will often gang up on the attacker.
- The dark markings around a meerkat's eyes act as sunglasses and help them to see even better.
- A meerkat's tail is about eight inches long, and it is used as a balancing tool to allow them to stand on their back legs.

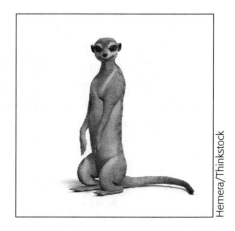

Hemera/Thinkstock

Activity Tips:

- Imagining sitting in a chair can help the understanding of proper body form and help keep the thighs parallel to the ground.
- The arms should be stretched as high as possible while sitting into the exercise so that the spine is straight.
- Any rounding of the back or sticking the hips out to the rear should be discouraged.

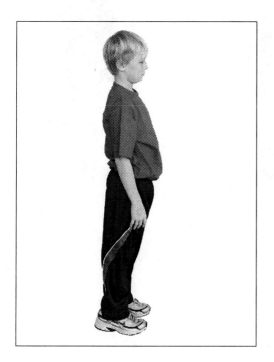
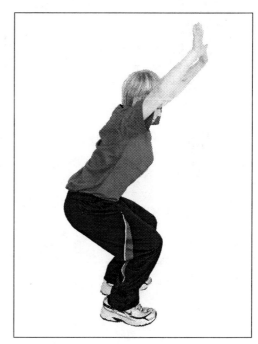

Flamingo

Animal Facts:

- A flamingo's pinkish-red color comes as a result of the algae that make up its diet.
- A flamingo's eye is larger than its brain.
- Flamingos are able to sit down by extending their legs backward.

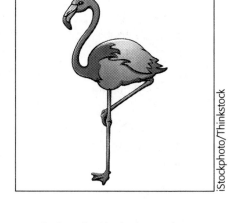

iStockphoto/Thinkstock

Activity Tips:

- The foot may be pressed into the inner thigh or leg to aid with balance.
- For better balance, the focus should be on a non-moving object in the line of vision.
- The key to success is to relax. The goal is not to muscle into being balanced.

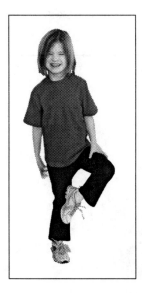 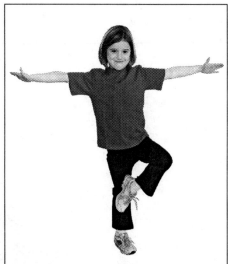 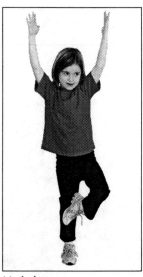

Variation

Brachiosaurus

Animal Facts:

- These dinosaurs were 85 feet long, 50 feet tall at the head, and weight about 90 tons.
- It was one of the dinosaurs to appear in the Jurassic Park movies.
- Its name means "arm lizard," as it front legs were longer than its back ones, giving it the appearance of a very large giraffe.

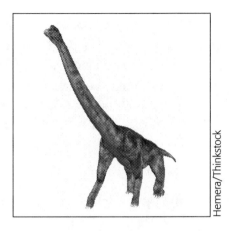

Hemera/Thinkstock

Activity Tips:

- The base leg needs to remain firm in order to maintain balance.
- The body weight should be on the foot, not the hand. Over time, attempts can be made to remove the hand from the ground.
- While some weight will be on the hand/fingers, the fingers should not bend backward.

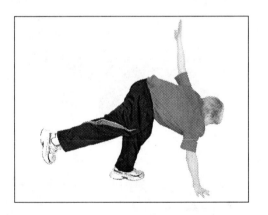
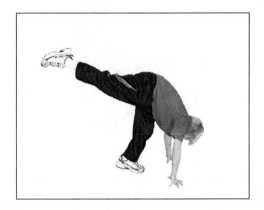

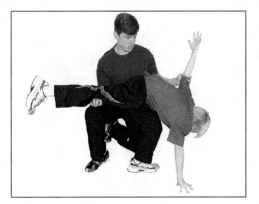

Tyrannosaurus Rex

Animal Facts:

- The T. rex had a head nearly five feet long with nine inch long serrated teeth.
- T. rex most likely ate his weight (16,000 pounds) in meat every week.
- As large as T. rex was, he had very short arms that were only about three feet long.

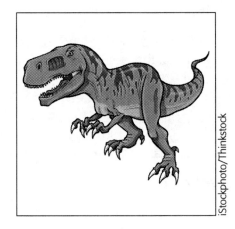

Activity Tips:

- The goal should be to open the chest throughout the exercise.
- A relaxed base leg and foot should be used as the primary tool for balance.
- The neck should remain in line with the spine; the head should not be allowed to droop.

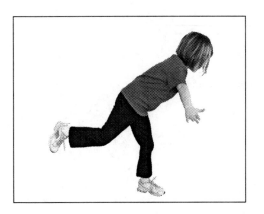
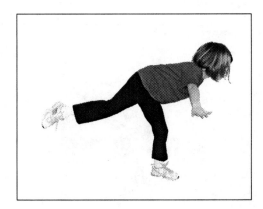

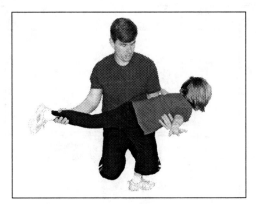

Bronco

Animal Facts:

- A bronco is a horse that is athletic, with a strong will, and a love for bucking.
- Some broncos can sell for up to $50,000.
- The state of Wyoming has used a bucking bronco on its license plates since 1936.

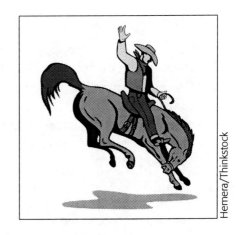

Activity Tips:

- The ball of the foot should be pushed toward the ceiling throughout the exercise.
- The body weight should be equally balanced between the arms and leg.
- The spine should be kept as straight and long as possible throughout the exercise.

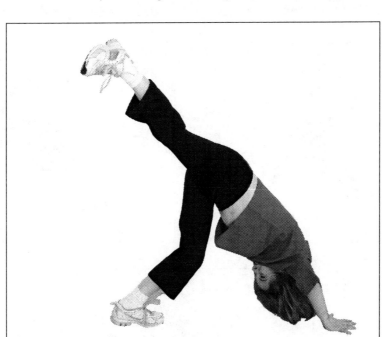

Praying Mantis

Animal Facts:

- Praying mantises are very difficult to see in the wild due to their excellent camouflage.
- The praying mantis is the only insect that can turn its head.
- Mantises have a hollow chamber within in them that helps them to detect their major predator: bats.

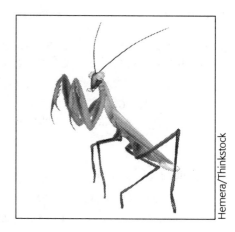

Activity Tips:

- The knees should be kept in line with the feet; as a rule, the toes should be visible.
- When in the correct position, the elbows should be pointing directly up and down.
- The shoulders, feet, and hips should be kept in a line throughout the exercise.

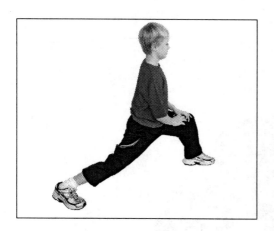
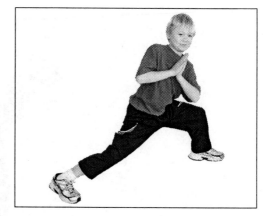

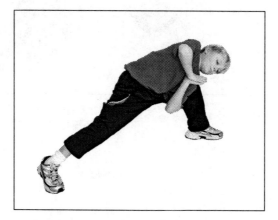

Cheetah

Animal Facts:

- Cheetahs are the fastest land animals, capable of running 70 mph.
- Cheetahs are, in some ways, more like dogs than cats; for example, they don't climb trees, they can't retract their claws, and they have long legs.
- Cheetahs do not roar like lions and tigers; instead, they make a sound like a bird chirping.

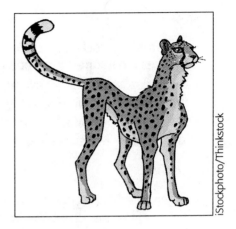

iStockphoto/Thinkstock

Activity Tips:

- The back should remain as straight as possible throughout the exercise.
- The hips should be relaxed so that the body weight can be used to lower into position.
- The knees should be kept in line with the feet; as a rule, the toes should be visible.

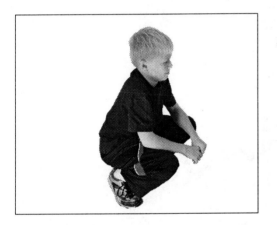
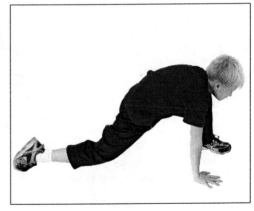

Peacock

Animal Facts:

- The word peacock only refers to the male, as females are referred to as peahens.
- Peacocks do more than just fan out their tails; they also vibrate them, which makes a rattling sound while showing off their colors.
- The peacock is the national bird of India.

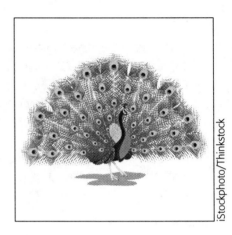

iStockphoto/Thinkstock

Activity Tips:

- When reaching back, the focus should be on opening the chest rather than bending backward.
- The toes are most important for balance. The toes should be used to grip the floor throughout the exercise.
- Holding breath should be discouraged. Breathing should be even and steady throughout.

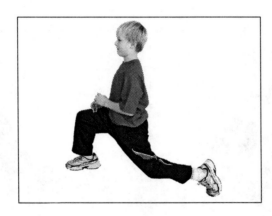

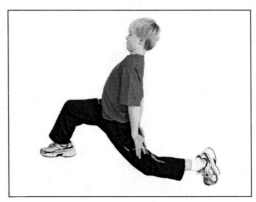

Pigeon

Animal Facts:

- Pigeons are capable of flying up to 50 mph.
- Pigeons have extraordinary homing skills, so good that they are used by many armies for delivering messages. In fact, they had a 98 percent success rate during World War II.
- Pigeons have been taught to use tools and to remember how to use those tools.

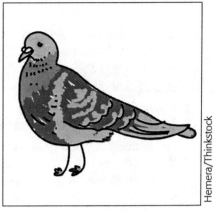

Activity Tips:

- The toes of the back foot should point directly backward.
- The hips should be level; one hip should not rise higher than the other.
- The arms should not be used to hold up the body. The body should be relaxed, as it is the body weight that will cause the stretch.

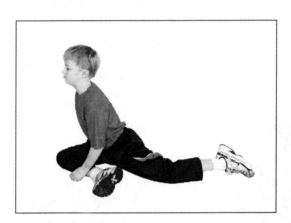

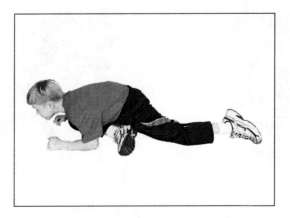

Swan

Animal Facts:

- Swans can be aggressive and have been known to bite; they are also powerful, so much so that their beating wings are capable of breaking a human arm.
- Swans build very large nests, some of which can measure 15 feet in diameter.
- Trumpeter swans are unique in that they are the largest of the aquatic birds, they are the rarest of all the swan species, and they mate for life.

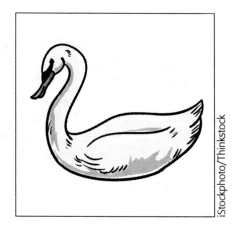

iStockphoto/Thinkstock

Activity Tips:

- When lowering to the ground, an attempt should be made to rest the chest on the front leg.
- Intensity can be increased by reaching forward with the arms after resting on the front leg.
- The torso should be kept level throughout; one side should not rest higher than the other.

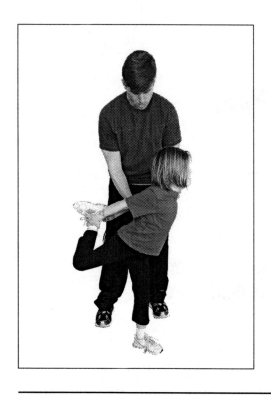
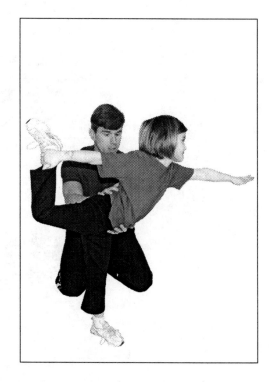

Butterfly

Animal Facts:

- Butterflies taste with their feet.
- Butterflies do not have mouths that allow for biting and chewing.
- Monarch butterflies migrate from the Great Lakes to the Gulf of Mexico—a distance of nearly 2,000 miles.

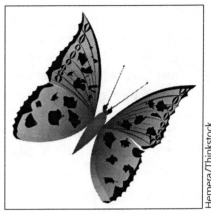

Hemera/Thinkstock

Activity Tips:

- The back must be kept straight throughout the exercise, even when leaning forward.
- The muscles of the outer hips, not the bouncing movement, should bring the legs to the floor.
- To vary the intensity, the distance between the feet and hips can be altered.

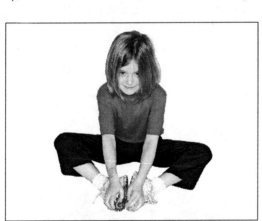

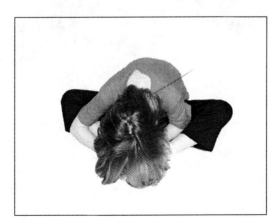

Anemone

Animal Facts:

- They have a round sucker that attaches them to rocks, and then they use tentacles to catch prey that swim past them.
- When it is frightened, it closes up its tentacles and looks like a blob of jelly.
- The anemone may be red, pink, or yellow and resemble flowers when tentacles are out.

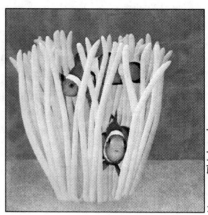

Hemera/Thinkstock

Activity Tips:

- All of the movements, whether side-to-side or forward, should come from the waist, not the neck.
- If the knees bend during the exercise, the participant should back off, reset, and then stretch again.
- Resistance from the muscles should be expected during this stretch; the focus should be to relax, work through it, and be patient.

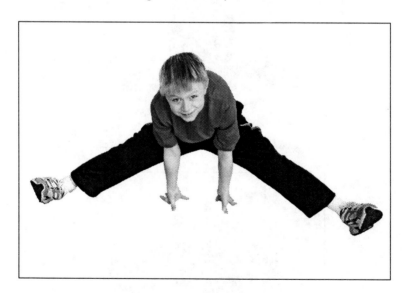

Turtle

Animal Facts:

- Sea turtles excrete salt from seawater through their eyes, giving them the appearance that they are crying.
- The leatherback turtle is the largest turtle, averaging 6.5 feet in length and weighing 1,500 pounds.
- Box turtles can eat so much that they will no longer fit inside their shells.

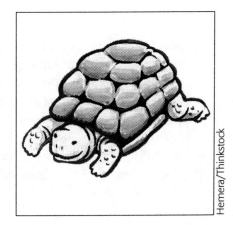

Hemera/Thinkstock

Activity Tips:

- To complete the exercise correctly, the participant must lead with the chest when bending forward into position.
- If the knees bend during the exercise, the participant should back off, reset, and then stretch again.
- The goal is to move slowly into the stretch and focus on breathing normally throughout the movement.

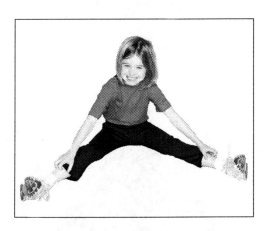

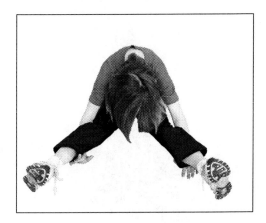

Ostrich

Animal Facts:

- Ostriches are the fastest two-legged animal in the world, capable of running up to 45 mph and maintaining that speed for 30 minutes.
- Ostriches are the largest living bird, standing up to 10 feet tall and weighing up to 350 pounds.
- An ostrich egg is the largest in the world; it is equivalent to 24 chicken eggs and takes nearly two hours to boil.

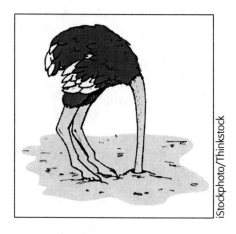

iStockphoto/Thinkstock

Activity Tips:

- Before beginning, the toes should point forward or slightly inward.
- Instead of trying to touch the forehead to the floor, the participant should put the top of the head as close to the floor as possible.
- The goal is to move slowly into the stretch, letting the weight of the body pull forward, then hold the stretch without bouncing.

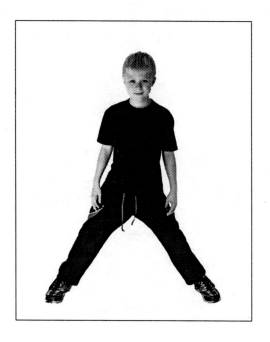
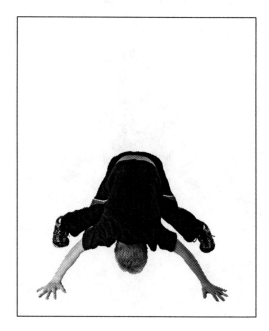

Cat

Animal Facts:

- A cat will almost never meow at another adult cat; that is a sound cats typically reserve for humans (or their mother when they are kittens).
- If a cat bites you after you rub its belly, it is probably doing so out of pleasure rather than anger.
- A cat's tail says a great deal about its mood: a wagging tail means a decision is imminent; a tail twitching at the tip is a sign of an angry cat; a low, fluffy tail is a frightened cat; a curved tail is a curious cat; and a high, arched tail is a sign of an impending cat fight.

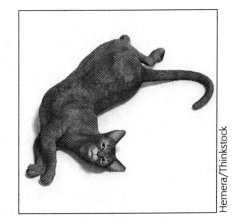

Hemera/Thinkstock

Activity Tips:

- The straight leg should not bend. If it does, the participant should back off a little and not stretch as deeply.
- The goal is to move into the twist slowly and gently; attempts to twist too forcefully should be discouraged.
- The holding of breath should be discouraged. The goal is to breathe normally throughout the exercise.

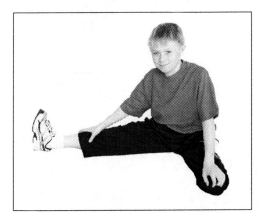
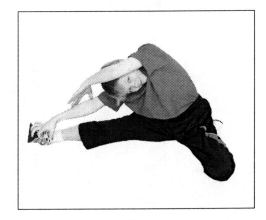

Eagle

Animal Facts:

- Eagles can fly up to 40 mph and can dive at over 100 mph.
- A bald eagle's wingspan is about eight feet wide.
- Eagles can even swim underwater using an overhand motion of their wings.

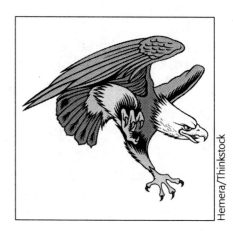

Hemera/Thinkstock

Activity Tips:

- The goal is to "fly" into the stretch by sweeping the arms back, then leaning into the stretch.
- While it should be avoided, it is okay if the heel comes off the ground.
- Most of the weight should be on the leg that is bent.

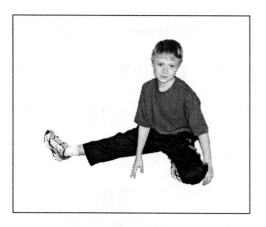

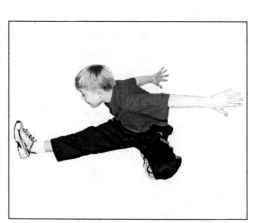

Rhinoceros

Animal Facts:

- A rhino's horn is made of tightly compacted hair.
- Rhinos are capable of running up to 45 mph; unfortunately they have poor eyesight and can only see 40 feet in front of them. Because of this, a group of rhinos are called a "crash."
- Unlike many animals, when a rhino is startled or afraid, it charges at the object scaring it, rather than running away.

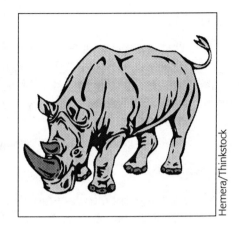

Hemera/Thinkstock

Activity Tips:

- The body must be balanced before beginning the exercise.
- The straightened leg should be grabbed as near to the foot as possible.
- The leg should not be pulled forcefully toward the body; instead, the body should lean backward to stretch the leg.

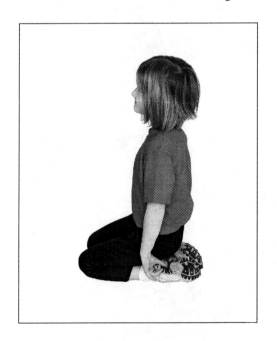

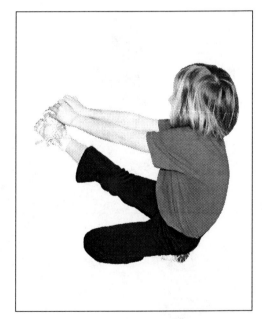

Ladybug

Animal Facts:

- Ladybugs use their feet to smell.
- Ladybugs produce a chemical substance that smells and tastes horrible. It prevents them from being eaten by birds and other predators.
- Ladybugs will clean themselves after a meal.

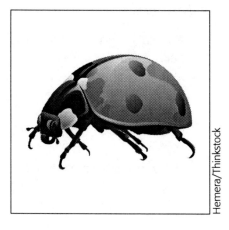

Hemera/Thinkstock

Activity Tips:

- Breathing should be normal, and the body weight should be used to pull into the stretch; the arms should not be used to pull.
- The back should remain straight throughout, and participants should lead with the chest.
- The goal for the exercise is not to touch the forehead to the thighs; instead, the aim should be to touch the chin to the shin.

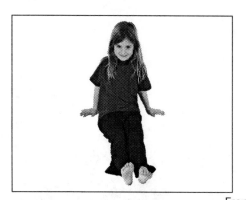
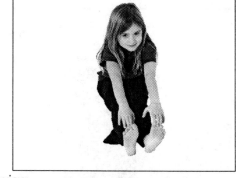

Front view

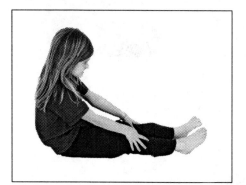
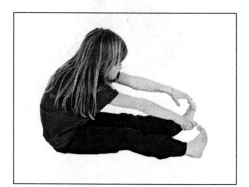

Side view

Itchy Dog

Animal Facts:

- Fleas are capable of jumping over 150 times their own length. That is like a human jumping 1,000 feet.
- Fleas have been around over 100 million years. That means that the dinosaurs had to deal with fleas as well.
- In one month, 10 fleas can produce 250,000 fleas.

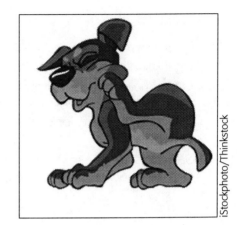

Activity Tips:

- Rather than the leg being pulled back into the stretch, the shoulder can be moved forward.
- The goal should be to move smoothly into the position, rather than jerking the leg backward.
- It is okay if the back rounds slightly while moving into the position.

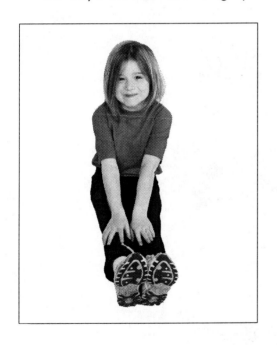
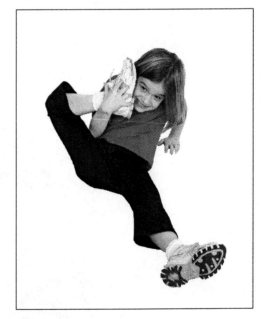

Otter

Animal Facts:

- Otters can hold their breath for up to eight minutes and swim 18 mph.
- Otters have special lenses on their eyes to make up for the distortion that occurs from looking at things underwater.
- Sea otters are rare in that they are one of a very few mammals that use tools.

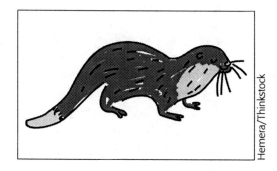

Hemera/Thinkstock

Activity Tips:

- The arms will need to lace between the legs for a good grip so as to remain in position throughout the exercise.
- Some "give and take" should be expected during the movement; in other words, participants will need to feel their way into the position.
- Once in position, both the feet and buttocks should be off the floor.

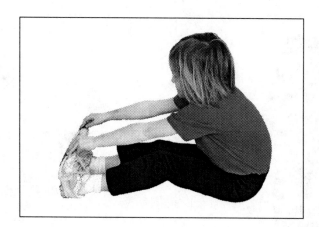

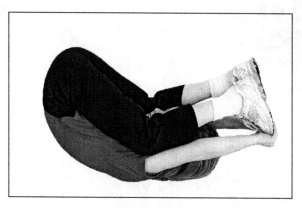

Arm and Shoulder Exercises

The arms and shoulders are among the most important muscles in the body. The arms and shoulders are so important because they control the position of the hands, thereby allowing interaction with the environment. The muscle of the arm that is targeted by these exercises is primarily the *triceps brachii*, the large muscle on the back of the arm. It is used for a great many different movements, including pushing motions as well as nearly any other motions that involve straightening the arm. The muscles of the shoulder that are targeted are many, including the *deltoids, pectoralis major, latissimus dorsi, teres major/minor, serratus anterior*, and *subscapularis*. These muscles are responsible for the myriad movements that occur at the shoulder, including flexion (lifting the arm to the front), extension (bringing it back down), abduction (lifting it up to the side), adduction (bringing it back down to the side), and all types of rotation. The shoulder muscles are used during all types of sports activities, including throwing (overhand and underhand), pulling, swinging, and other activities of play and sport. Building strength in the shoulders is important in keeping the joint healthy. As the bones of the shoulder joint lack a good fit (unlike those in the hip), it is at risk for dislocation or other injury. Having strong muscles around the area of the shoulder gives the joint an extra level of protection and stability that it would otherwise lack. The shoulder must hold a delicate balance between strength and flexibility, and that is what the exercises in this chapter do. They help build the strength in the shoulders without increasing their size dramatically. In this way, it is possible to gain the benefits of extra stability in the shoulders without losing the important range of motion it provides.

Walking Stick

Animal Facts:

- They are the longest insects in the world, some measuring over 21 inches in length.
- The walking stick's body so closely resembles a leaf and twigs that it uses that as its major form of defense against predators.
- The walking stick's scientific name, Phasmida, is a Greek word meaning apparition. With a name like that, it is no wonder that these insects seem to disappear like a ghost.

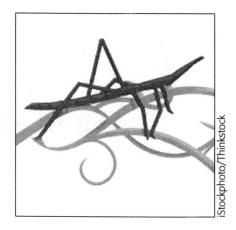

iStockphoto/Thinkstock

Activity Tips:

- The torso and hips should form a line and remain tight during the exercise.
- Throughout the exercise, the shoulders should be directly over the hands while the gaze is kept downward.
- Normal breathing should be maintained throughout the exercise.

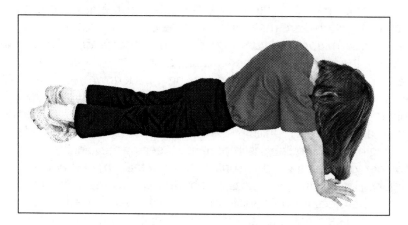

Water Strider

Animal Facts:

- They are able to walk on water because they have very small, water-repellent hairs that hold air bubbles. It is these bubbles that allow them to skate across the water.
- They use their three sets of legs in different ways: their front set is used for grabbing prey; the second set is used as paddles; and the third set is used as a rudder for steering.
- Water striders communicate with each other by sending ripples across the water.

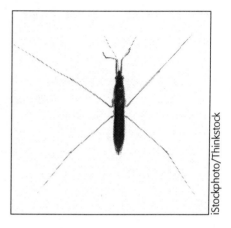

iStockphoto/Thinkstock

Activity Tips:

- The arms and legs should be kept straight and at a 45-degree angle to the body.
- The body should remain tight while keeping the hips from drooping in the middle.
- The focus should be kept on preventing the hands and feet from getting too close to one another.

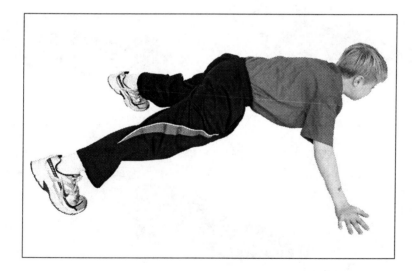

Woodpecker

Animal Facts:

- A woodpecker can peck up to 20 times per second.
- Woodpeckers are able to hold onto trees because two of their toes face the front and two toes face the back.
- Woodpeckers have larger-than-normal neck and shoulder muscles compared to most other birds.

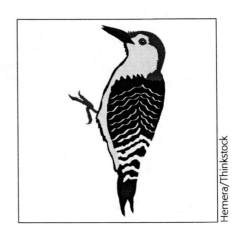

Hemera/Thinkstock

Activity Tips:

- The body should move as a single unit throughout the exercise.
- The focus must be kept on the ground between the hands.
- The body should be lowered until the chest touches the ground.

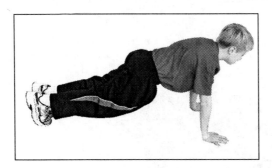
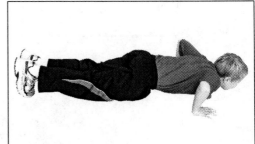
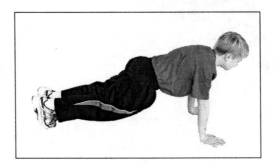

Scorpion

Animal Facts:

- Placing a tiny drop of liquor on a scorpion will make it crazy, and it will sting itself to death.
- Scorpions give birth to live babies, and the mother will carry them around on her back.
- Scorpions are able to live for a month with only water.

Activity Tips:

- The body should move as a single unit during the exercise; it should not sag in the middle.
- The leg should be lifted as high as possible before bending.
- The back should not excessively arch during the exercise.

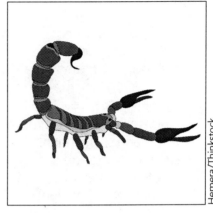

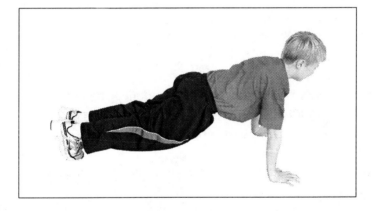

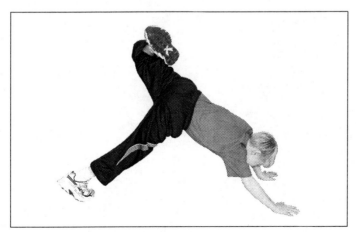

Wolf

Animal Facts:

- Wolf puppies love to play, just like dog puppies. They will roll around with each other and play with "toys" like bones, feathers, sticks, or anything they can find with which to amuse themselves.

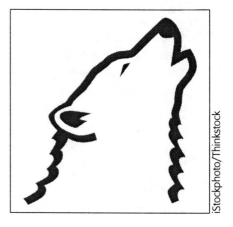

- Wolves communicate through body language. The leaders, the Alpha male and female, are the biggest and strongest and hold their tails the highest. The lowest members, the Omega male and female, keep their tails between their legs. When angry, they stick their ears up and show their teeth; when suspicious, they squint and pull their ears back; when afraid, they flatten their ears against their head; when playful, they will dance and prance and put their back end up in the air.

- Wolves also "talk." They howl, bark, growl, chirp, and squeak, and mother wolves even make a whimpering noise that calms their puppies.

Activity Tips:

- The following should brush on the ground during the exercise (in order): nose, chin, chest, and abdomen.
- The intensity can be changed by pushing straight back at the end rather than retracing the path.
- The shoulders should be kept over the hands as much as possible.

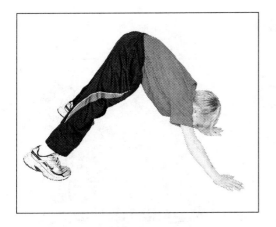 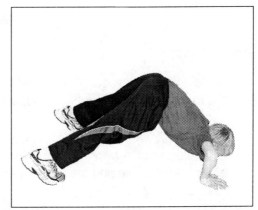

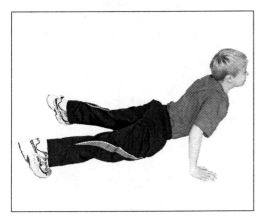 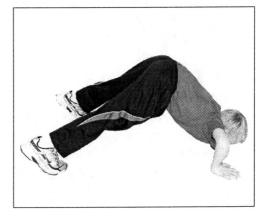

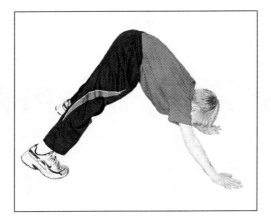

Walrus

Animal Facts:

- Walruses are very social animals and generally like to hang out and "chat" in groups that can number over one hundred.
- A walrus's whiskers, which give it the appearance of having a moustache, are extremely sensitive and are used for detecting food underwater.
- You can tell how old a walrus is by counting the rings in a cross-section of one of his tusks, much like you can determine the age of a tree by counting its rings.

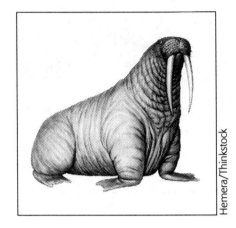

Hemera/Thinkstock

Activity Tips:

- The arms should be used to pull up while keeping the points of the hips on the ground. The hips should not swing during the movement.
- In order to ensure correct technique, the insteps should be kept on the ground; the balls of the feet should not be used to push.
- The arms should be slightly bent while moving forward.

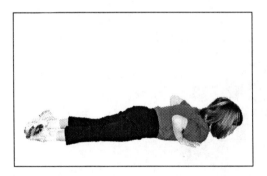
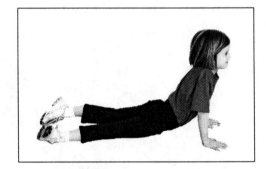
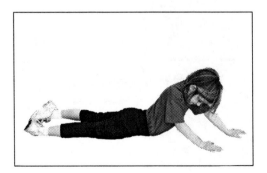
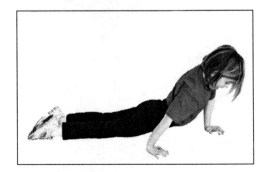

Alligator

Animal Facts:

- The largest alligator ever was found in Louisiana, and it was 19'2".
- Alligators are capable of sprinting up to 20 mph over short distances.
- An alligator can go through between 2,000 and 3,000 teeth in a lifetime.

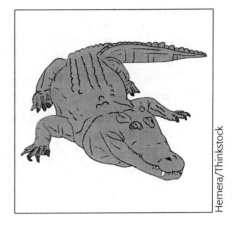

Hemera/Thinkstock

Activity Tips:

- The body must be kept tight and moving as a unit throughout the exercise.
- The same side arm and leg should be moving simultaneously.
- The only points of contact with the floor are the palms and the balls of the feet.

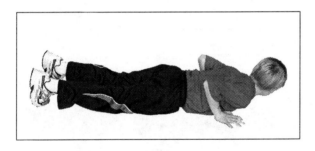

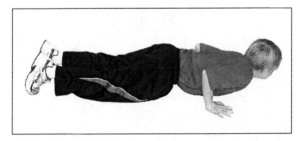

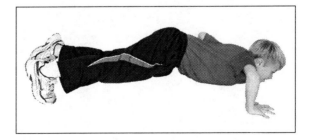

Katydid

Animal Facts:

- Katydid antennae are two to three times the length of their body. This allows them to find their way around in the dark.
- Katydids hear through slits in their front legs.
- There are about 2000 katydid species, each of which has its own unique "song."

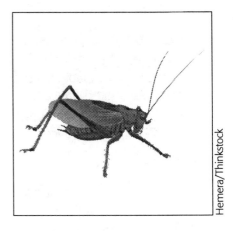

Activity Tips:

- The knee should strive to touch the back of the arm.
- The focus is to stretch as far as possible with the arm in front.
- In order to maintain proper form, the knee should be kept pointing up throughout the exercise.

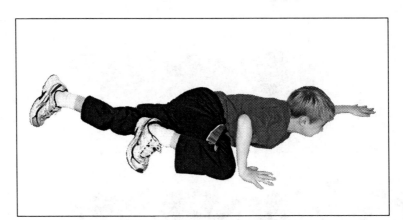

Black Widow

Animal Facts:

- The black widow is considered the most venomous spider in North America.
- Only the females are dangerous, males and infants are harmless.
- Eggs sacs can hold between 25 and 900 eggs.

Activity Tips:

- In order to move smoothly, the leg should be brought as close to the arm as possible.
- The body must stay very low to the ground with only the palms and feet touching the floor.
- The body should remain parallel to the floor; the hips should not point up in the air.

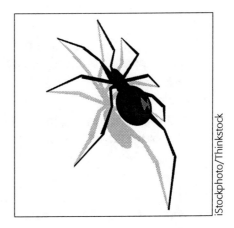

iStockphoto/Thinkstock

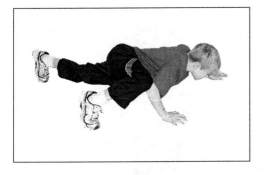 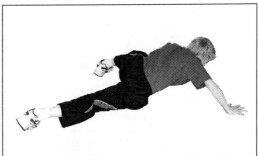

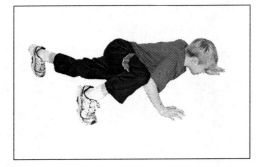

Cow

Animal Facts:

- Cows drink about a bathtub full of water and eat 40 pounds of food per day.
- Cows produce 90 percent of the milk in the world.
- A cow will produce almost 200,000 glasses of milk throughout her life.

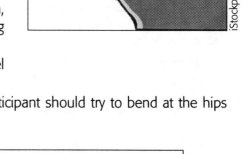

Activity Tips:

- In order to get the most out of the stretch, both of the knees should be pointing forward.
- If the hands cannot touch in back, a towel may be used to connect them.
- Once the final position is achieved, the participant should try to bend at the hips and rest the throat on the top knee.

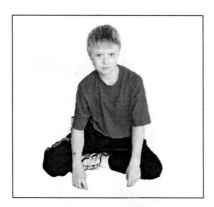

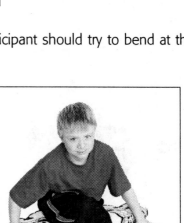

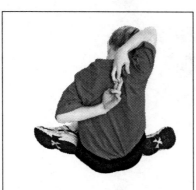

Rear view

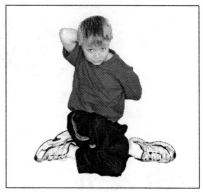

Front view

Lizard

Animal Facts:

- Some lizards can change colors in response to their mood.
- The largest lizard in the world is the Komodo dragon at 10 feet long and up to 350 pounds.
- While they have poor hearing and sight, their senses of taste and smell allow them to detect food up to five miles away.

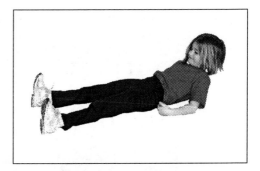

Activity Tips:

- Only the forearms and heels should be in contact with the floor.
- A constant push with the hips up toward the ceiling should be maintained throughout the movement.
- The legs must be kept straight so as not to push off with the heels and propel forward.

iStockphoto/Thinkstock

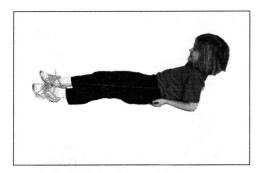

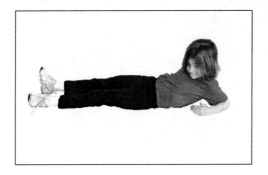

Crab

Animal Facts:

- The Japanese spider crab is the largest crab in the world, with a body width of 15 inches, a 12-foot leg span, and a weight of 50 pounds.
- Crabs eat nearly anything they can get their claws on, including: plants, fish, carrion (dead animals), or even their own young.
- Coconut crabs have pincers strong enough to crack a coconut. Oddly enough, this type of crab cannot swim and will drown if put in the water.

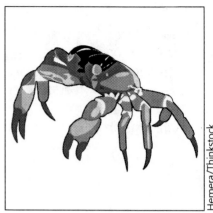

Hemera/Thinkstock

Activity Tips:

- The belly button should be pushed up throughout the movement to keep a "tabletop" position.
- A relaxing position should be found for the head. This position must not allow the neck to bend too much in either direction.
- The feet should stay in line with the knees and the shoulders in line with the hands throughout the movement.

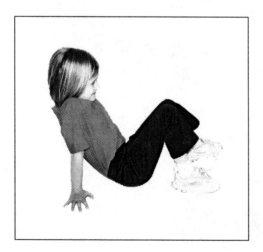
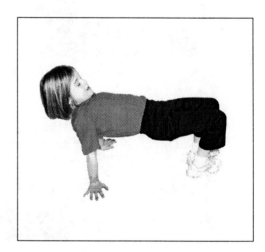

Stegosaurus

Animal Facts:

- Stegosaurus means "roof reptile." It was so named because it had plates on its back that were approximately three feet long that were thought to overlap slightly like roofing tiles.
- A full-grown Stegosaurus, while measuring about 30 feet long, nine feet tall, and weighing between four and six tons (about the size of a bus), had a brain about the size of a golf ball.
- It is theorized that Stegosaurus had a second brain in its hip, which was responsible for controlling the back end of its body.

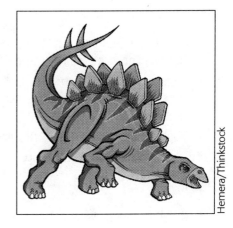

Hemera/Thinkstock

Activity Tips:

- A constant push should be maintained with the hips up toward the ceiling throughout the movement.
- The hips should not droop in the middle as the leg is lifted.
- The lifted leg should be kept as straight as possible, but it should not be the primary focal point.

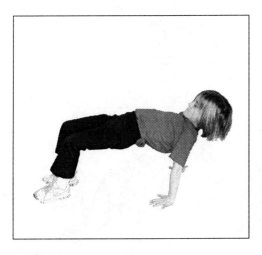 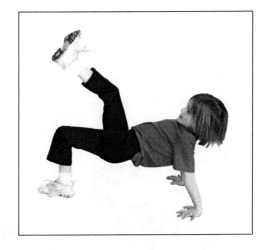

Hungry Dog

Animal Facts:

- Greyhounds can run up to 45 mph, a speed that can reach after only three strides.
- Dogs only sweat from the bottoms of their feet; the only way they discharge heat is by panting.
- Dogs yawn as a sign of contentment.
- Dogs have no sense of time.

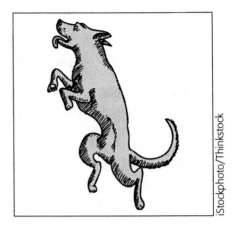

iStockphoto/Thinkstock

Activity Tips:

- The hips should be pushed upward toward the sky when sliding a leg under the body.
- One leg should always be swinging under the body; the movement does not involve stepping over one leg with another.
- The exercise involves constant motion, like a spinning top.

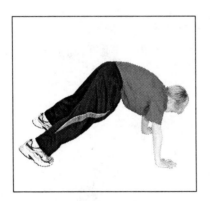
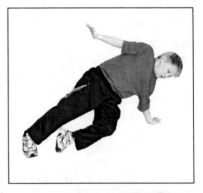

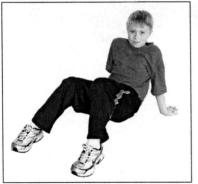
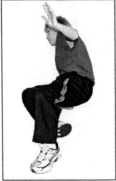
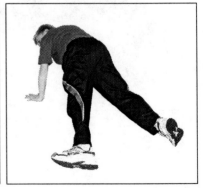

Slug

Animal Facts:

- A slug has four noses.
- A slug's slime is very important; it acts as a defense mechanism because its poor taste keeps predators away, it is a natural anaesthetic, it prevents water loss, and it allows them to fit into tight places, stick to steep surfaces, and even hang from a ceiling.
- Slugs have about 25,000 teeth and use them to eat twice their weight in food a day.

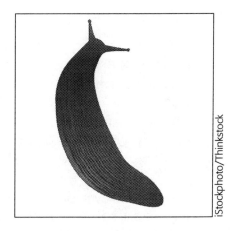

iStockphoto/Thinkstock

Activity Tips:

- The body should be as stretched out as possible before the movement.
- Only the arms should be used to pull forward; the hips should not rock and the feet should not push.
- The knees can bend to make the exercise easier.

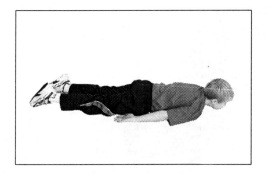
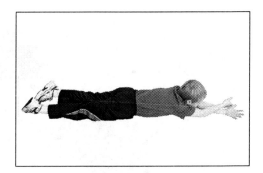
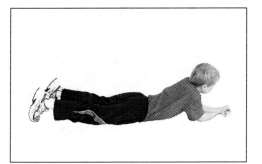
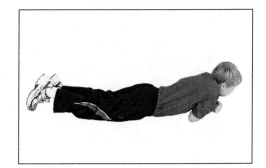

Caterpillar

Animal Facts:

- Ladybugs are one of the most common predators of the caterpillar.
- Caterpillars are typically striped with an orange head.
- They are cannibals and will eat one another until only one remains on an ear of corn.

Activity Tips:

- During the movement, the body should not push backward toward the hamstrings; rather, it should push upward toward the ceiling.
- The forearms need to be flat on the floor with the head hanging in a comfortable position.
- It is okay if the heels are not flat on the floor.

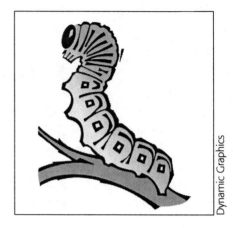

Dynamic Graphics

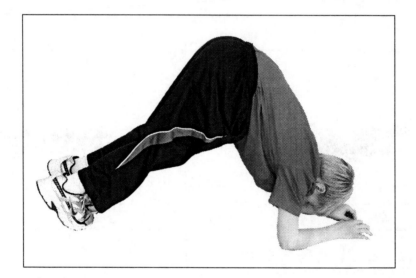

Stretching Dog

Animal Facts:

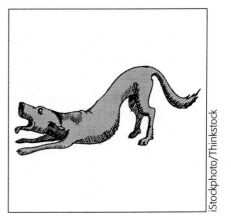

- Dogs, in general, have a sense of smell one hundred thousand to a million times more sensitive than a human's; a scent hound such as a bloodhound, basset hound, or beagle has a sense of smell one to 10 million times more sensitive.
- While dogs are able to see in color, they do not see it as vividly as we do; instead, their vision is like ours at twilight.
- Dog nose prints may be used to identify dogs just as fingerprints are used to identify humans.

Activity Tips:

- During the movement, the body should not push backward toward the hamstrings; rather, it should push upward toward the ceiling.
- It is okay if the heels are not flat on the floor.
- The movement should be thought of as a fluid thing, rather than a static stretch.

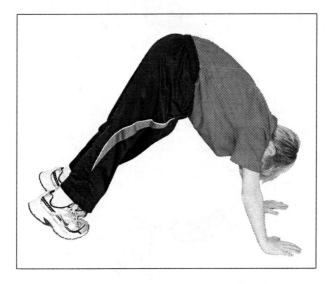

Giraffe

Animal Facts:

- Giraffes can grow to be 19 feet tall, weigh over 1,600 pounds, and have a 16-inch tongue.
- The word giraffe come from an Arabic word meaning "the tallest of all."
- Giraffes sleep deeply for only a few minutes at a time.

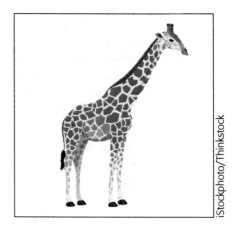

Activity Tips:

- For safety, the leg should be lifted, and not swung, into position.
- Even with the leg in the air, the hips should continue to push upward toward the ceiling.
- Breathing should be kept constant throughout the exercise, timing the exhale with the lifting of the leg.

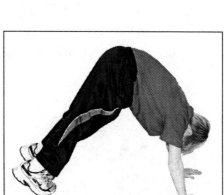

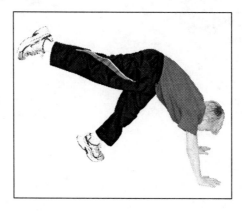

Bear

Animal Facts:

- Bears are as intelligent as the great apes and possess excellent long-term memories.
- Fit bears are able to run up to 30 mph over short distances.
- Bears typically treat humans as other bears. Unfortunately, that is a little rougher than humans are accustomed to being handled.

Activity Tips:

- The arms and legs should be kept relaxed. It will make it easier to find the rhythm of the movement.
- The head should only be lifted enough to see.
- The arms and legs should be moved like a gallop, fluid with the movement.

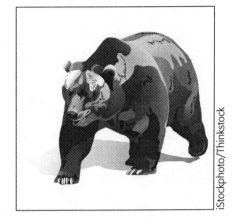

iStockphoto/Thinkstock

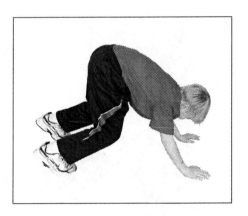 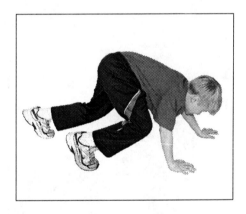

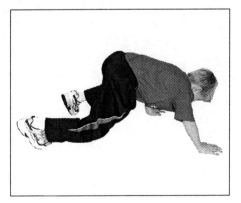

Parakeet

Animal Facts:

- The parakeet is one of the most popular pet birds in the United States.
- Parakeets come in many different colors, such as light blue, yellow, dark green, purple, white, or any combination of those colors.
- Parakeets can be trained to sit on your finger, and some can even be taught to talk.

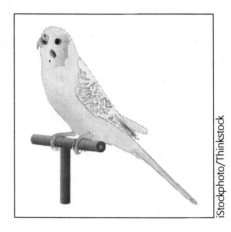

Activity Tips:

- The knees should be pulled tightly into the chest throughout the exercise.
- If the arms are too short, fingertips, fists, or even blocks can be used.
- Comfort is key; participants should find the best arm position for their body.

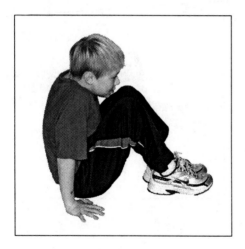
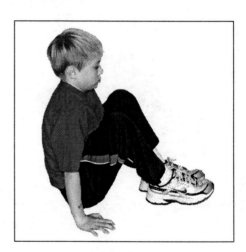

Crow

Animal Facts:

- Crows are considered to be the most intelligent of all the bird species.
- Crows are able to mimic other sounds and can associate sounds with specific events.
- A group of crows is referred to as a murder.

Activity Tips:

- In order to maintain balance, the eyes should be focused on the ground.
- For proper form, the knees must be kept on the outside of the upper arms; the knees should not rest on the back of the arms.
- Only the arms should be used; participants should not balance on the head like a tripod.

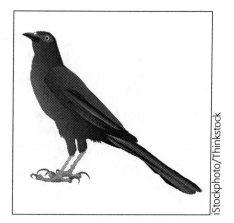

iStockphoto/Thinkstock

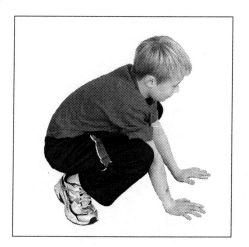
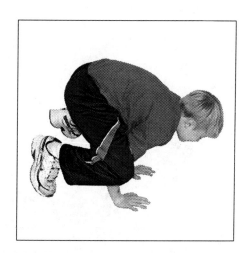

Frog

Animal Facts:

- The earliest frogs appeared nearly 190 million years ago, and it is believed they developed the ability to jump to avoid becoming lunch for a dinosaur.
- The largest frog, the Goliath frog, can grow to nearly 15 inches and weigh eight pounds.
- Frogs do not drink water; instead, they absorb it through their skin.

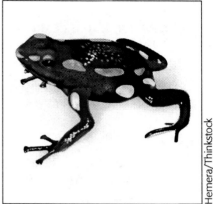

Hemera/Thinkstock

Activity Tips:

- The fingers can be spread apart for better balance.
- Once off the ground, the big toes should try to touch together.
- Participants should take their time; the movement should not be rushed or "jumped" into.

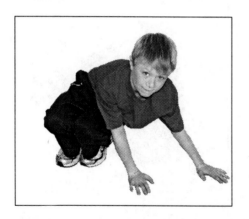
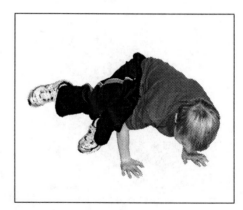
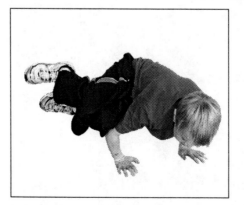

Peregrine Falcon

Animal Facts:

- Peregrine falcons are capable of level flight at over 60 mph, but during a dive, they can reach speeds of up to 200 mph.
- Peregrine falcons catch their prey in flight by hitting it with a half-closed talon and then catching it before it hits the ground.
- Falcons have a protruding, cone-shaped nostril that allows them to breathe during dives; jet designers copied this design so that they could make the jet engines work at high speeds.

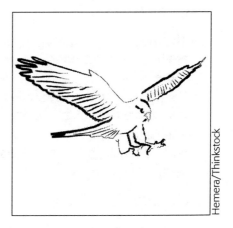

Hemera/Thinkstock

Activity Tips:

- Only the arms should be used; participants should not balance on their head.
- The extended leg may be either straight or bent, depending on balance.
- Participants should only slide into the final position to mimic a diving falcon once they are comfortable with Crow.

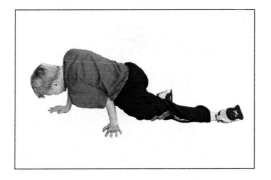

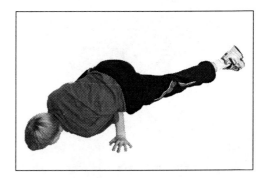

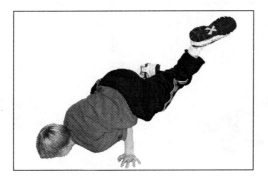

Bird of Paradise

Animal Facts:

- The bird of paradise uses brightly colored feathers and elaborate dances to attract mates.
- They are considered by some to be the most impressive birds in the world.
- The Great Bird of Paradise is 18 inches long with 24-inch plumes extending from its wings.

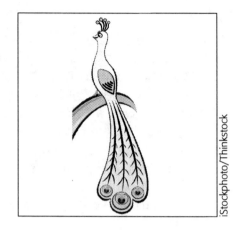

iStockphoto/Thinkstock

Activity Tips:

- The forearms should be kept together; they should not flare out.
- It is vital for stability that the elbows are kept in contact with the abdomen during the exercise.
- This exercise should be avoided if it hurts the wrists.

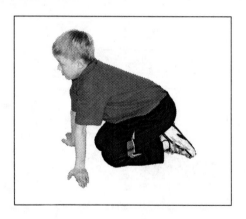
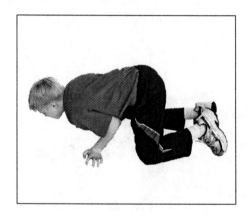
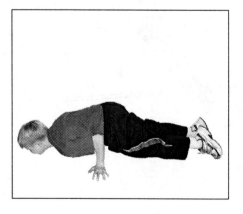
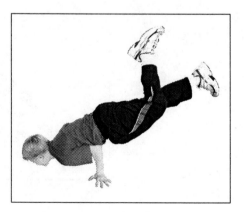

Gorilla

Animal Facts:

- Although gorillas cannot talk, they are capable of understanding spoken language and have been taught to perform sign language.
- Gorillas are extremely intelligent and share many emotions with humans, such as: love, hate, fear, grief, pride, generosity, and jealousy.
- Gorillas will laugh when tickled and cry when hurt.

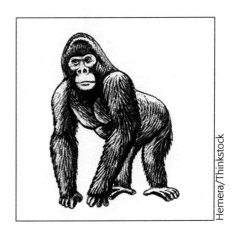

Hemera/Thinkstock

Activity Tips:

- As with Parakeet, fingertips, fists, or blocks may be used if the arms are too short.
- The feet should swing completely past the hands so that the exercise is finished with the feet in front of the hands.
- To be successful, the knees should be pulled tightly into the chest during the swing.

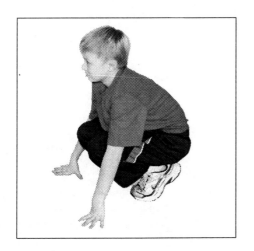 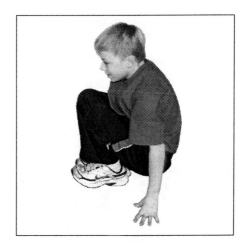

Appendix:

Sample Exercise Programs

Under the Sea

- Narwhal
- Catfish
- Puffer Fish
- Shark
- Shrimp
- Otter
- Anemone
- Turtle

Creepy Crawlies

- Caterpillar
- Inchworm
- Scorpion
- King Cobra
- Slug
- Black Widow
- Sidewinder
- Eel
- Tarantula

A Bug's Life

- Walking Stick
- Water Strider
- Roly-Poly
- Praying Mantis
- Ladybug
- Click Beetle

Dino-Might

- Brachiosaurus
- Tyrannosaurus Rex
- Lizard
- Crab
- Stegosaurus
- Ankylosaurus

On Safari

- Lion
- Gorilla
- Tiger
- Cheetah
- Rhinoceros
- Giraffe
- Meerkat

Old MacDonald

- Rabbit
- Itchy Dog
- Duck
- Cow
- Horse
- Wolf
- Stretching Dog
- Bronco

Up, Up, and Away

- Butterfly
- Pigeon
- Eagle
- Flying Squirrel
- Woodpecker
- Parakeet
- Crow
- Peregrine Falcon
- Bird of Paradise

References

1. Nemet D, Berger-Shemesh E, Wolach B, Eliakim A. (2006). A combined dietary-physical activity intervention affects bone strength in obese children and adolescents. *International Journal of Sports Medicine*. Aug; 27(8): 666-71.

2. Manias K, McCabe D, Bishop N. (2006). Fractures and recurrent fractures in children; varying effects of environmental as well as bone size and mass. *Bone*. Sep; 39(3): 652-7.

3. Ahrens W, Bammann K, de Henauw S, Halford J, Palou A, Pigeot I, Siani A, Sjostrom M. (2006). Understanding and preventing childhood obesity and related disorders—IDEFICS: a European multilevel epidemiological approach. *Nutrition, Metabolism, and Cardiovascular Disease*. May; 16(4): 302-8.

4. Wearing SC, Hennig EM, Byrne NM, Steele JR, Hills AP. (2006). The impact of childhood obesity on musculoskeletal form. *Obesity Review*. May; 7(2): 209-18.

5. Raitakari OT, Juonala M, Viikari JS. (2005). Obesity in childhood and vascular changes in adulthood: insights into the Cardiovascular Risk in Young Finns Study. *International Journal of Obesity*. Sep; 29 Suppl 2: S101-4.

6. Freedman DS, Dietz WH, Tang R, Mensah GA, Bond MG, Urbina EM, Srinivasan S, Berenson GS. (2004). The relation of obesity throughout life to carotid intima-media thickness in adulthood: the Bogalusa Heart Study. *International Journal of Obesity and Related Metabolic Disorders*. Jan; 28(1): 159-66.

7. Skilton MR, Celermajer DS. (2006). Endothelial dysfunction and arterial abnormalities in childhood obesity. *International Journal of Obesity*. Jul; 30(7): 1041-9.

8. Misra A. (2000). Risk factors for atherosclerosis in young individuals. *Journal of Cardiovascular Risk*. Jun; 7(3): 215-29.

9. Mitsnefes MM. (2006). Hypertension in children and adolescents. *Pediatric Clinics in North America*. Jun; 53(3): 493-512.

10. Rosenberg B, Moran A, Sinaiko AR. (2005). Insulin resistance (metabolic) syndrome in children. *Panminerva Medica*. Dec; 47(4): 229-44.

11. Serdula MK, Ivery D, Coates RJ, Freedman DS, Williamson DF, Byers T. (1993). Do obese children become obese adults? A review of the literature. *Preventative Medicine*; 22.

12. Whitaker RC, Wright JA, Pepe MS, Seidel KD, Dietz WH. (1997). Predicting obesity in young adulthood from childhood and parental obesity. *New England Journal of Medicine*. Sep; 337(13).

13. Kotani K, Nishida M, Yamashita S, Funahashi T, Fujioka S, Tokunaga K, Ishikawa K, Tarui S, Matsuzawa Y. (1997). Two decades of annual medical examinations in Japanese obese children: do obese children grow into obese adults? *International Journal of Obesity and Related Metabolic Disorders*. Oct; 21(10).

14. Goran MI. (2001). Metabolic precursors and effects of obesity in children: a decade of progress, 1990-1999. *American Journal of Clinical Nutrition*. Feb; 73(2): 158-71.

15. Daniels SR. (2006). The consequences of childhood overweight and obesity. *The Future of Children*. Spring; 16(1): 47-67.

16. Flodmark CE. (2005). The happy obese child. *International Journal of Obesity*. Sep; 29 Suppl 2: S31-3.

17. Stunkard AJ, Faith MS, Allison KC. (2003). Depression and obesity. *Biological Psychiatry*. Aug 1; 54(3): 330-7.

18. Young-Hyman D, Tanofsky-Kraff M, Yanovski SZ, Keil M, Cohen ML, Peyrot M, Yanovski JA. (2006). Psychological status and weight-related distress in overweight or at-risk-for-overweight children. *Obesity*. Dec; 14(12): 2249-58.

19. Hasler G, Pine DS, Kleinbaum DG, Gamma A, Luckenbaugh D, Aidacic V, Eich D, Rossler W, Angst J. (2005). Depressive symptoms during childhood and adult obesity: the Zurich Cohort Study. *Molecular Psychiatry*. Sep; 10(9): 842-50.

20. Zeller MH, Modi AC. (2006). Predictors of health-related quality of life in obese youth. *Obesity*. Jan; 14(1): 122-30.

21. Warschburger P. (2005). The unhappy obese child. *International Journal of Obesity*. Sep; 29 Suppl 2: S127-9.

22. Banis HT, Varni JW, Wallander JL, Korsch BM, Jay SM, Adler R, Garcia-Temple E, Negrete V. (1988). Psychological and social adjustment of obese children and their families. *Child Care, Health, and Development*. May-Jun; 14(3): 157-73.

23. Robinson S. (2006). Victimization of obese adolescents. *Journal of School Nursing*. Aug; 22(4): 201-6.

24. Hayden-Wade HA, Stein RI, Ghaderi A, Saelens BE, Zabinski MF, Wilfley DE. (2005). Prevalence, characteristics, and correlates of teasing experiences among overweight children vs. non-overweight peers. *Obesity Research*. Aug; 13(8): 1381-92.

25. Neumark-Sztainer D, Falkner N, Story M, Perry C, Hannan PJ, Mulert S. (2002). Weight-teasing among adolescents: correlations with weight status and disordered eating behaviors. *International Journal of Obesity and Related Metabolic Disorders*. Jan; 26(1): 123-31.

26. Keery H, Boutelle K, van den Berg P, Thompson JK. (2005). The impact of appearance-related teasing by family members. *Journal of Adolescent Health*. Aug; 37(2): 120-7.

27. Eisenberg ME, Neumark-Sztainer D, Story M. (2003). Associations of weight-based teasing and emotional well-being among adolescents. *Archives of Pediatric and Adolescent Medicine*. Aug; 157(8): 733-8.

28. Clement K, Boutin P, Froguel P. (2002). Genetics of obesity. *American Journal of Pharmacogenomics*. 2(3): 177-87.

29. Herbert A, Gerry NP, McQueen MB, Heid IM, Pfeufer A, Illig T, Wichmann HE, Meitinger T, Hunter D, Hu FB, Colditz G, Hinney A, Hebebrand J, Koberwitz K, Zhu X, Cooper R, Ardlie K, Lyon H, Hirschhorn JN, Laird NM, Lenburg ME, Lange C, Christman MF. (2006). A common genetic variant is associated with adult and childhood obesity. *Science*. Apr 14; 312(5771): 279-83.

30. Harvard University. (2001). Weight loss and gain. *Harvard Health Letter*. 26(5): 1-3.

31. Parsons TJ, Power C, Logan S, Summerbell CD. (1999). Childhood predictors of adult obesity: a systematic review. *International Journal of Obesity and Related Metabolic Disorders*. Nov; 23 Suppl 8: S1-107.

32. Burke V, Beilin LJ, Dunbar D. (2001). Family lifestyle and parental body mass index as predictors of body mass index in Australian children: a longitudinal study. *International Journal of Obesity and Related Metabolic Disorders*. Feb; 25(2): 147-57.

33. Maffeis C, Talamini G, Tato L. (1998). Influence of diet, physical activity and parents' obesity on children's adiposity: a four-year longitudinal study. *International Journal of Obesity and Related Metabolic Disorders*. Aug; 22(8): 758-64.

34. Whitaker RC, Deeks CM, Baughcum AE, Specker BL. (2000). The relationship of childhood adiposity to parent body mass index and eating behavior. *Obesity Research*. May; 8(3): 234-40.

35. Campbell K, Waters E, O'Meara S, Summerbell C. (2001). Interventions for preventing obesity in childhood. A systematic review. *Obesity Reviews*. Aug; 2(3): 149-57.

36. Salinsky E. (2006). Effects of food marketing to kids: I'm lovin' it? Issue Brief: National Health Policy Forum. Aug; 15(814): 1-16.

37. Faith MS, Kerns J. (2005). Infant and child feeding practices and childhood overweight: the role of restriction. *Maternal and Child Nutrition*. Jul; 1(3): 164-8.

38. Anderson PM, Butcher KE. (2006). Childhood obesity: trends and potential causes. *The Future of Children*. Spring; 16(1): 19-45.

39. Uauy R, Diaz E. (2005). Consequences of food energy excess and positive energy balance. *Public Health Nutrition*. Oct; 8(7A): 1077-99.

40. He M, Irwin JD, Sangster-Bouck LM, Tucker P, Pollet GL. (2005). Screen-viewing behaviors among preschoolers parents' perceptions. *American Journal of Preventive Medicine*. Aug; 29(2): 120-5.

41. Caroli M, Argentiere L, Cardone M, Masi A. (2004). Role of television in childhood obesity prevention. *International Journal of Obesity and Related Metabolic Disorders*. Nov; 28 Suppl 3: S104-8.

42. Strasburger VC. (2006). Children, adolescents, and advertising. *Pediatrics*. Dec; 118(6): 2563-9.

43. Gable S, Chang Y, Krull JL. (2007). Television watching and frequency of family meals are predictive of overweight onset and persistence in a national sample of school-aged children. *Journal of the American Dietetics Association*. Jan; 107(1): 53-61.

44. Coon KA, Tucker KL. (2002). Television and children's consumption patterns. A review of the literature. *Minerva Pediatrica*. Oct; 54(5): 423-36.

45. Viner RM, Cole TJ. (2005). Television viewing in early childhood predicts adult body mass index. *Journal of Pediatrics*. Oct; 147(4): 429-35.

46. Hancox RJ, Milne BJ, Poulton R. (2004). Association between child and adolescent television viewing and adult health: a longitudinal birth cohort study. *Lancet*. Jul 17-23; 364(9430): 257-62.

47. Must A, Tybor DJ. (2005). Physical activity and sedentary behavior: a review of longitudinal studies of weight and adiposity in youth. *International Journal of Obesity*. Sep; 29 Suppl 2:S84-96.

48. Flynn MA, McNeil DA, Maloff B, Mutasingwa D, Wu M. (2006). Reducing obesity and related chronic disease risk in children and youth: a synthesis of evidence with 'best practice' recommendations. *Obesity Review*. Feb; 7 Suppl 1: 7-66.

49. Lamonte MJ, Blair SN. (2006). Physical activity, cardiorespiratory fitness, and adiposity: contributions to disease risk. *Current Opinions in Clinical Nutrition and Metabolic Care*. Sep; 9(5): 540-6.

50. Yang X, Telama R, Viikari J, Raitakari OT. (2006). Risk of obesity in relation to physical activity tracking from youth to adulthood. *Medicine and Science in Sports and Exercise*. May; 38(5): 919-25.

51. Nelson MC, Gordon-Larsen P. (2006). Physical activity and sedentary behavior patterns are associated with selected adolescent health risk behaviors. *Pediatrics*. Apr; 117(4): 1281-90.

About the Author

Tony Kemerly, Ph.D., is an associate professor of exercise science and the chair of the Department of Exercise and Sport Science at High Point University, in High Point, North Carolina. Kemerly teaches in both the undergraduate and graduate programs at HPU. His courses include human anatomy, biomechanics, strength and conditioning, health behavior change, and physical activity and obesity. His books include *Biomechanics: Analyzing Human Movement* and *Taekwondo Grappling Techniques*. Kemerly is a 1996 graduate of McNeese State University in health promotion and a 1998 graduate of Louisiana Tech University in exercise science. He earned a Ph.D. in exercise science from the University of Mississippi in 2001.